BE HEART SMART

...the HCF way to a healthy heart.

by James W. Anderson, M.D.

A Publication of
The HCF Nutrition
Research Foundation, Inc.

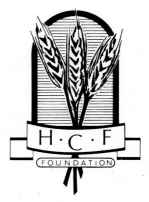

James W. Anderson, M.D.
with
Nancy Gustafson, M.S., R.D.

Many thanks for the invaluable assistance provided by
Cynthia Chandler Kennedy, M.S., R.D.
and Susan Eviston, R.D.

Typography and Design by
CRYSTAL PUBLICATION SERVICES
Lexington, Kentucky
Ed Puterbaugh, Creative Director

Artwork by
RON BELL ILLUSTRATIONS
Lexington, Kentucky

Distributed by
The HCF Nutrition Research Foundation, Inc.
Box 22124
Lexington, KY. 40522
(606) 276-3119

First Printing January 1989

ISBN: 0-922859-00-0

CONTENTS

1

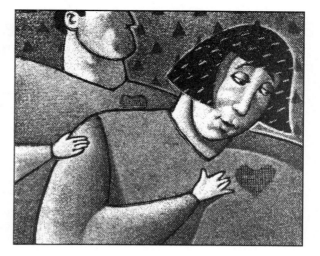

HEART TO HEART

E ach year about one million Americans die of heart attack or stroke — that's one person every 30 seconds. One of every two Americans will die of heart and blood vessel diseases, and one in every four living persons suffer some form of these diseases. Heart and blood vessel diseases kill more of us than all other causes of death combined, with heart attack topping the list.

Heart and blood vessel diseases, also called cardiovascular diseases, affect the young and old. One in five cardiovascular disease deaths occur in persons under age 65. Forty-five percent of all heart attack victims are under age 65, and males ages 55 to 64 years old experience more heart attacks than any other age group. If you are male, your chances of suffering a heart attack before age 60 are one in five.

WHAT IS CARDIOVASCULAR DISEASE?

Cardiovascular disease refers to a group of diseases affecting the heart (cardio) or blood vessels (vascular). One of the most common cardiovascular diseases is **high blood pressure**, a condition where the heart must pump harder than normal to circulate blood through the body. This strains the heart and wears and tears on

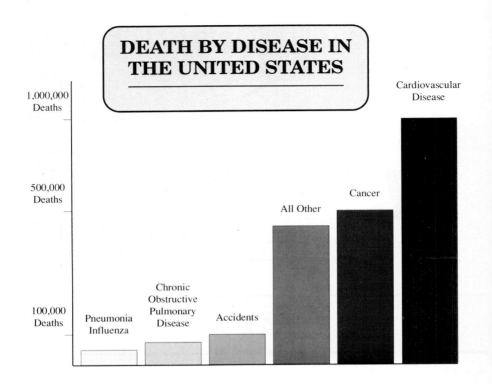

DEATH BY DISEASE IN THE UNITED STATES

the blood vessels, contributing to other forms of cardiovascular disease such as hardening of the arteries, heart attack and stroke.

Hardening of the arteries, or **atherosclerosis**, also greatly contributes to cardiovascular disease deaths. Hardening of the arteries occurs when fatty deposits of cholesterol and other material build up in the inner lining of the blood vessels, making them less flexible.

These deposits can begin as early as childhood and grow gradually throughout adulthood, squeezing off blood flow to vital organs in the body. Eventually these deposits can totally block blood flow or break off and become lodged in another blood vessel. If blood flow to the heart stops, a **heart attack** occurs. If blood flow to the brain stops, a **stroke** occurs. In either case blood flow to the organ is inadequate for proper functioning, and tissue begins to die.

Sometimes our bodies give us warning signs of impending heart attack or stroke. As blood vessels to the heart narrow and blood supply becomes inadequate, some people experience chest pain, also called **angina**. Angina can be the first symptom of a heart attack, or it can occur by itself.

If blood supply to the brain is inadequate or temporarily blocked, some people experience mini-strokes, or **transient ischemic attacks**. Temporary dizziness or loss of speech, vision, or other body functions characterize these mini-strokes, which often signal an impending major stroke.

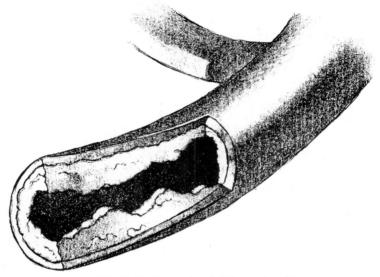

The Fatty Deposits of Atherosclerosis.

With **congestive heart failure,** another form of cardiovascular disease, the heart is weakened and cannot pump efficiently. Fluid often builds up in the ankles, legs, lungs and other tissues. High blood pressure and atherosclerosis can weaken the heart, as can rheumatic heart disease, an infection that begins with strep throat.

Proper eating and living habits beginning in childhood can prevent or greatly lessen the severity of most cardiovascular diseases. However, changing to healthy habits at any age will reduce death and disability from these diseases.

WHAT CAUSES CARDIOVASCULAR DISEASE?

The same set of risk factors apply to most heart and blood vessel diseases. Some of these factors are within your control; some are not.

The older you get, the more likely you are to develop some type of cardiovascular disease. Males are also more likely than females to develop cardiovascular disease. Risk for heart attack, for example, is much lower in women than men. After menopause heart attack risk for women increases, but never equals that of men.

Black individuals are more susceptible to cardiovascular disease than white individuals because they develop high blood pressure more frequently. Having a family history of heart attack, stroke, or other cardiovascular disease also raises your risk.

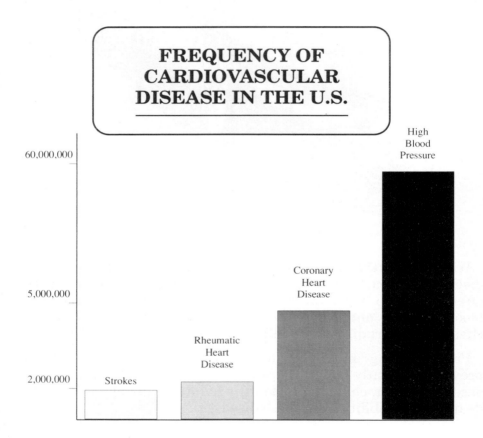

FREQUENCY OF CARDIOVASCULAR DISEASE IN THE U.S.

You can control several risk factors for cardiovascular disease. Too much fat and cholesterol in the blood contributes to hardening of the arteries and greatly increases your risk of heart attack or stroke. High blood pressure strains the heart and speeds up hardening of the arteries. Cigarette smoking raises blood pressure,

Chapter 1 HEART TO HEART

strains the heart, and promotes hardening of the arteries and clot formation.

Obesity, inactivity, and high blood sugar or diabetes also increase risk for cardiovascular disease, both independently and through their effects on blood cholesterol and blood pressure. In some individuals, a stressful lifestyle may also contribute to cardiovascular disease.

RISK FACTORS FOR HEART DISEASE AND STROKE

BEYOND CONTROL

Age	Gender
Race	Heredity

CONTROLLABLE

Blood cholesterol	Blood pressure
Triglyceride level	Cigarette smoking
Weight	Inactivity
Diabetes	Stress

Each of the major risk factors under our control for heart disease (high blood cholesterol, high blood pressure, and cigarette smoking) more than triple the risk of heart attack or stroke. If two or three of these major risk factors apply, your risk increases up to 15-fold. The greater number of risk factors present, the more your risk multiplies.

WHAT CAN I DO TO PREVENT CARDIOVASCULAR DISEASE?

Americans are already taking steps to prevent heart disease and stroke. We are eating better, exercising more, and living more healthful lifestyles than we did 10 to 20 years ago. These steps are paying off. Between 1965 and 1985 the death rate from heart disease declined 40 percent. We have come a long way, but we still have a long way to go.

The steps to a healthy heart and reduced cardiovascular disease risk include proper eating habits, maintenance of a healthy body weight, regular exercise, non-smoking, effective stress management, and regular health care visits. A small percentage of people may also need medication to control risk factors such as high blood pressure or high blood fat levels.

If you are young, you have much to gain by being heart smart. Fatty streaks can start in the blood vessels even during childhood, and blood vessel damage is already well under way by middle age for many Americans. But it is never too late to begin heart smart habits. These habits can strengthen the heart and reduce its work load. New evidence shows that some hardening of the arteries may even be reversible.

The chapters in this book discuss the major risk factors for heart and blood vessel diseases and give practical guidelines on how to control them. By following these steps, you will greatly reduce your chances of heart attack, stroke, and other cardiovascular diseases. You will also look better, feel better, and enjoy improved health and well-being.

2

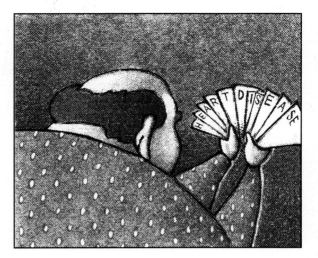

THE BIG FAT DEAL

Medical researchers hotly debated relationships between amount and type of fat eaten, blood fat levels, and risk of heart disease until recently.   The consensus is now clear: high blood cholesterol levels greatly increase risk for cardiovascular disease, and a high fat and cholesterol diet, such as the typical American diet, contributes to high blood cholesterol levels.

Countries with the highest fat and cholesterol intakes also have the highest rates for heart disease, and America ranks among the top. More than one-half of Americans have high blood cholesterol levels, according to new standards set by medical experts. High levels of cholesterol and other fats in the blood clog the vessels, causing hardening of the arteries and sometimes triggering a heart attack or stroke.

WHAT ARE BLOOD FATS?

Cholesterol and triglycerides are two blood fats you have probably heard of. Cholesterol is a waxy, fat-like substance found only in animal tissue. The body needs some cholesterol to make hormones, cell membranes, and other body substances. Too much cholesterol

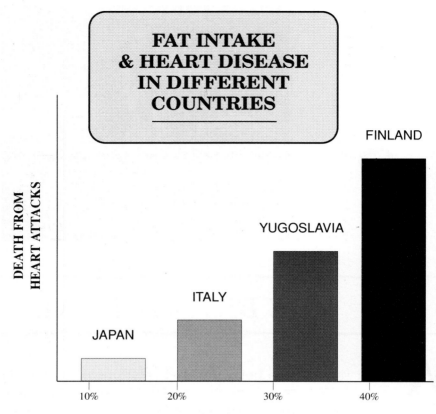

**FAT INTAKE
& HEART DISEASE
IN DIFFERENT
COUNTRIES**

DEATH FROM HEART ATTACKS

FINLAND

YUGOSLAVIA

ITALY

JAPAN

10%   20%   30%   40%

FAT IN DIET (% of calories)

in the body, however, can narrow blood vessels and greatly increase risk for heart disease.

Triglyceride refers to the chemical storage form of fat in the body. When we eat more calories than we need for growth and main-tenance of tissue, the excess calories are converted to triglycerides and stored in our fat cells.

High blood cholesterol levels accelerate hardening of the arteries and promote heart attack and stroke. High blood triglyceride levels often accompany high blood cholesterol levels; recent evidence shows high blood triglyceride levels independently increase risk for cardiovascular disease.

Cholesterol and other fats are carried in the blood in tiny pack-ages of fat and protein called lipoproteins. One type of lipoprotein, the low-density lipoprotein (LDL), is particularly prone to clog blood vessels and contribute to heart disease or stroke. LDL contains mostly fat and cholesterol and little protein. High LDL levels are usually associated with a high total cholesterol level.

Another type of lipoprotein, the high-density lipoprotein (HDL), contains mostly protein and helps remove excess cholesterol from the body. High HDL levels can actually reduce risk of heart disease or stroke.

A third type of lipoprotein, the very-low-density lipoprotein (VLDL), is a dumping vehicle for excess calories eaten from fat, sugar and alcohol. VLDL contains high levels of triglyceride and may also promote cardiovascular disease.

WHAT RAISES BLOOD FAT LEVELS?

Many factors affect our blood fat levels, including age, sex and heredity. The foods we eat also affect our blood fat levels.

Excess calories from fat, sugar or alcohol stimulate the body to make more triglycerides. While its true that our own bodies make most of the cholesterol circulating in the blood, a high intake of cholesterol and fat in the diet raises blood cholesterol levels.

Cholesterol is only found in animal food. Plant foods contain no cholesterol. **Appendix I lists the cholesterol content of many common foods**. Egg yolks and organ meats such as liver contain high amounts of cholesterol. Lean red meats, poultry and shellfish contain moderate amounts of cholesterol. Fish and dairy products in the amounts commonly consumed contain smaller amounts of cholesterol.

A certain type of fat called **saturated fat** is particularly prone to raise blood cholesterol levels. Animal fats contain mostly saturated fats, as do a few plant fats, including palm, palm kernel, and coconut oil.

HOW DO I KNOW IF MY BLOOD FAT LEVELS ARE TOO HIGH?

Your doctor can order simple blood tests to determine your cholesterol and/or triglyceride levels. Blood triglycerides are usually measured after an overnight fast. If your blood fat levels are high, your doctor may also want you to fast overnight for a more detailed blood test to determine levels of specific blood fats like HDL and LDL cholesterol.

Risk for heart disease sharply rises with blood cholesterol levels over 200 mg/dl (milligrams per deciliter — the units of measurement for blood cholesterol). Therefore, a desirable blood cholesterol level is less than 200 mg/dl, or around 180 mg/dl. A desirable blood triglyceride level is less than 250 mg/dl,some experts recommend that the triglycerides be below 150 mg/dl.

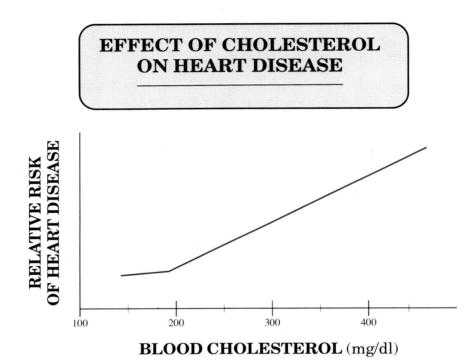

EFFECT OF CHOLESTEROL ON HEART DISEASE

RELATIVE RISK OF HEART DISEASE

100   200   300   400

BLOOD CHOLESTEROL (mg/dl)

More than one-half of middle-aged Americans have high blood cholesterol levels. About 10 percent of Americans have high blood triglyceride levels, which are frequently accompanied by high blood cholesterol levels.

In the past, many physicians considered a cholesterol level of even 260 to 280 mg/dl to be normal. We now know that these levels are much too high. In fact, most heart attacks occur in people with cholesterol levels of 210 to 265 mg/dl.

If you do not know what your blood cholesterol level is, ask your doctor. If your blood cholesterol is less than 200 mg/dl, have it checked at least every two years. If you have other heart disease risk factors such as high blood pressure, have your cholesterol level

TARGET BLOOD CHOLESTEROL

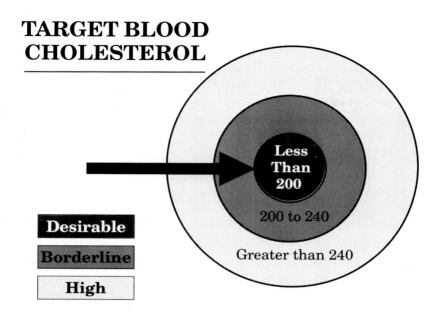

Desirable

Borderline

High

Less Than 200

200 to 240

Greater than 240

Target Blood Cholesterol (in mg/dl)

TARGET BLOOD TRIGLYCERIDES

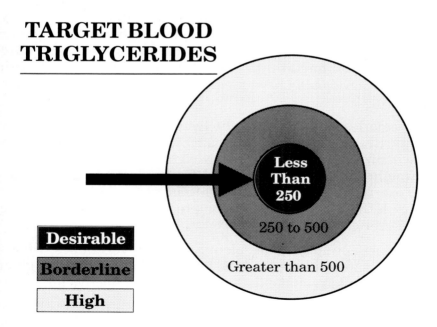

Desirable

Borderline

High

Less Than 250

250 to 500

Greater than 500

Target Blood Triglycerides (in mg/dl)

checked every year. If your cholesterol level is 200 to 240 mg/dl, you should take steps to lower it and also have it checked yearly.

If your cholesterol is over 240 mg/dl, you should have detailed blood fat analysis to determine LDL and HDL cholesterol levels. You will also require close medical and dietary follow-up to be sure these blood fat levels return to a more healthy range. Your doctor will probably want to recheck your blood fat levels one to two months after you change to a more healthy diet and lifestyle habits.

HOW CAN I LOWER MY BLOOD FAT LEVELS?

If you have high blood fat levels, the best time to lower them is now. The younger you are, the more you stand to gain.

For every one percent you lower your cholesterol level, you reduce your risk for heart disease two percent. For example, suppose your cholesterol level was 250 mg/dl and you lowered it to 200 mg/dl through healthy eating and regular exercise. You reduced your cholesterol by 20 percent and reduced your risk for heart disease by 40 percent.

Most people can lower their blood fat levels significantly if they follow the simple guidelines in this book for weight control, regular exercise and proper eating habits. Regular doctor visits and blood fat checks are also important. A small percentage of people with high blood fat levels may need medication to bring the levels back to normal.

Excess calories and body weight feed high blood fat levels by pumping extra fat into our systems. Blood triglycerides usually increase in direct proportion to body weight. If you are overweight, losing weight will often lower blood fat levels 10 to 20 percent. Regular exercise helps you lose weight and also raises levels of the protective HDL cholesterol while helping to lower the damaging LDL cholesterol.

Heart smart eating includes plenty of fruits, vegetables, whole-grain breads and cereals, and dried beans and peas. Foods high in a type of fiber called soluble fiber are especially effective for lowering blood fat levels.

Oat products, dried beans and peas, and psyllium fiber supplements contain generous amounts of soluble fiber. Avoid foods high in cholesterol such as egg yolks, organ meats, or high-fat red meats. Limit use of fats and oils, avoiding saturated fats such as butter, lard, palm, palm kernel or coconut oil whenever possible. Use less meat and choose the leanest cuts, emphasizing poultry and fish as animal protein sources. Select low-fat dairy products and indulge in high-fat, sugary desserts only on special occasions. Some people with high blood triglycerides may also need to avoid or limit alcohol.

Heart smart eating is easy if you make the changes gradually ...and it is healthy for the entire family. A high-carbohydrate, high-fiber and low-fat diet drops blood fat levels 20 to 30 percent, reducing risk for heart disease 40 to 60 percent.

KNOW YOUR FATS

(Test your nutrition knowledge by responding to the following TRUE/FALSE questions. Answers are at the end of the chapter.)

1. Only meats contain saturated fats.
2. The body needs some cholesterol.
3. Cottage cheese contains less fat than cream cheese.
4. Frying foods is okay as long as you use a polyunsaturated oil.

WHO NEEDS MEDICATION?

Most people can control their blood fat levels with diet and lifestyle changes; less than twenty percent of people with high blood fat levels need medication.

If your blood cholesterol level is high, give proper diet and exercise a diligent try for four to six weeks, then have your cholesterol level rechecked. If your level is still above 200 mg/dl, you may need to make further diet changes, such as lowering your fat intake to 20 percent of calories or adding more fiber.

If your blood cholesterol level is still above 240 mg/dl three to six months after a change of diet, your doctor may suggest you add medication to your cholesterol-lowering program. If you have other risk factors for heart disease, your doctor may decide to start medication if your cholesterol is above 200 mg/dl.

If your blood triglycerides are seriously high (above 2,000 mg/dl), or if they remain above 500 mg/dl after three months of healthy eating, exercise and weight management habits, you may need triglyceride-lowering medication.

Your doctor will recommend the blood-fat-lowering medication that is right for you. Some medications only lower blood cholesterol, some lower only blood triglycerides, and a few do both. Some come in the form of pills and others in powder you mix with water or fruit juice.

MEDICATIONS THAT LOWER BLOOD FATS

Medication	Lowers Cholesterol	Lowers Triglycerides	Side Effects
Colestipol	Yes	No	Constipation, bloating, increased gas production, nausea
Cholestyramine	Yes	No	Same as Colestipol
Clofibrate	Sometimes	Yes	Well-tolerated
Gemfibrozil	Sometimes	Yes	Well-tolerated
Lovastatin	Yes	No	Well-tolerated
Nicotinic Acid	Yes	Yes	Flushing of the skin, stomach irritation, abnormal liver tests, diarrhea
Probucol	Yes	No	Diarrhea

Medications such as cholestyramine and colestipol have been used for a long time and have a proven safety record. A new medication called Lovastatin appears to be even more effective than these medications with fewer side effects, but its long-term safety has not been fully tested. Most medications lower blood fat levels 10 to 30 percent. Lovastatin appears to lower blood cholesterol levels 25 to 45 percent.

Psyllium, the main active ingredient in certain laxatives such as Metamucil, also lowers blood cholesterol about 15 percent. Psyllium has few side effects and is very safe for long-term use. For some people, taking two or three doses of sugar-free Metamucil or other psyllium fiber products daily might be a reasonable compromise between diet alone and diet and medication.

Medication should be added to a diet and lifestyle program when necessary, not substituted for it. Proper diet enhances the effectiveness of cholesterol- or triglyceride-lowering medications; a poor diet works against them.

Without a healthy diet and lifestyle, medications to lower blood fat levels will have little effect. You will also miss out on other benefits of proper diet and exercise habits, such as improved health, looks and well-being; a higher energy level; and reduced risk for other diseases.

ANSWERS TO "KNOW YOUR FATS" QUIZ:

1. **FALSE**. Saturated fat, the type of fat linked to raising blood cholesterol levels, is found mainly in animal products but is also found in palm oil and coconut oil. Watch for these oils on the ingredient list of many snack foods and mixed dish items. Avoid these oils if you are trying to limit saturated fats.

2. **TRUE**. Cholesterol is needed by the body to make cell membranes, hormones and other substances. But the body can make all the cholesterol it needs. The liver makes about 1,000 milligrams (mg) daily. This means we need to limit the amount of cholesterol we put into our body from foods such as meat, fats and dairy products.

3. **TRUE**. Cream cheese is over 90% fat, almost all fat! Cottage cheese varies in the amount of fat it contains, but skim milk based cottage cheese contains as little as 2% fat. Regular cottage cheese has 4% fat so choose low-fat or uncreamed varieties. You can also rinse regular cottage cheese in a strainer to reduce the fat. Cream cheese is not a high quality nutritional food.

4. **FALSE**. Frying foods with any type of oil will greatly increase the calories in your meals. Of course, if you are eating fried foods it is better to choose polyunsaturated or monounsaturated oils to fry in but they contain the same number of calories as the saturated fats. You save no calories by choosing unsaturated fats although they are a better choice for keeping the blood vessels clean.

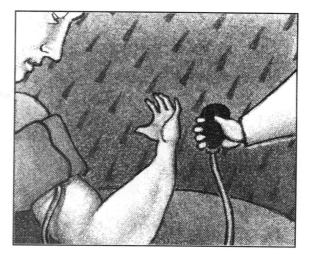

3

TAKING THE PRESSURE OFF

High blood pressure, or "hypertension", is the most common form of cardiovascular disease in the United States. It affects nearly 60,000,000 adults and 3,000,000 children, or almost 25% of the American population. People who are elderly, obese, black or use oral contraceptives are more likely to develop high blood pressure.

Doctors often call high blood pressure the silent killer because it causes no symptoms. Many people aren't even aware they have high blood pressure and therefore do not seek treatment.

High blood pressure greatly increases your risk for heart attack and stroke. The higher your blood pressure, the greater your risk. Even a mild blood pressure elevation raises your risk for all major forms of cardiovascular disease, especially when added to other risk factors such as cigarette smoking or high blood cholesterol. High blood pressure puts additional strain on your heart and adds to wear and tear on the blood vessels.

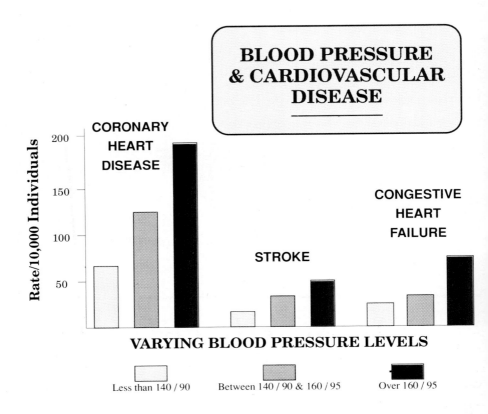

BLOOD PRESSURE & CARDIOVASCULAR DISEASE

CORONARY HEART DISEASE

CONGESTIVE HEART FAILURE

STROKE

Rate/10,000 Individuals

200

150

100

50

VARYING BLOOD PRESSURE LEVELS

Less than 140 / 90   Between 140 / 90 & 160 / 95   Over 160 / 95

WHAT IS HIGH BLOOD PRESSURE?

Blood pressure is the force the pumping heart creates as it pushes blood against the blood vessel walls. Blood pressure is measured in millimeters of mercury (mm Hg), and is read as two numbers. The upper number, called the systolic pressure, is the force of blood against the vessel walls when the heart is beating. The lower number, called the diastolic pressure, is the force of blood against the vessel walls between heartbeats.

Health professionals define high blood pressure in different ways, but usually define it as a systolic blood pressure 140 mm Hg or more and/or a diastolic pressure of 90 mm Hg or more. Because blood pressure fluctuates throughout the day, doctors must document high blood pressure with several readings over time.

With high blood pressure, the heart works harder to pump blood through the vessels. When we become excited, for example, the small blood vessels constrict, forcing the heart to pump harder to squeeze blood through. The heart must also work harder when the blood vessels become tight and inelastic, as with hardening of the arteries. When we eat more salt than needed, excess fluid can accumulate in tissues, making the heart work harder.

Extra strain on the heart can eventually enlarge it and interfere with efficient pumping. The extra force on the blood vessel walls increases wear and tear and contributes to hardening of the arteries. To help avoid these problems and greatly reduce your risk for cardiovascular disease, try to keep your blood pressure less than 120/80 mm Hg.

WHAT CAUSES HIGH BLOOD PRESSURE ?

An underlying health problem such as a kidney abnormality, adrenal gland tumor, or defect of the aorta causes high blood pressure in about five percent of cases. Causes are less clear in the remaining 95% of cases, but doctors know that certain factors contribute to high blood pressure.

The older we grow, the more likely we are to develop high blood pressure. Black Americans also develop high blood pressure two to three times more often than white Americans. If other members of our family have high blood pressure, we are more likely to have high blood pressure. Some women also get high blood pressure during pregnancy or while taking oral contraceptives.

Many factors that foster high blood pressure are beyond our control, while others are within our power to change. Blood pressure and body weight usually go together. If you are overweight, your chances of developing high blood pressure increase. Likewise, lack of physical activity tends to raise blood pressure. In some individuals, eating excess salt promotes fluid retention and blood vessel constriction, raising blood pressure. Continual stress can also contribute to high blood pressure in some individuals.

People who consume large amounts of caffeine or alcohol may be at risk for high blood pressure. Though not fully understood, the minerals calcium, magnesium and potassium appear to affect blood pressure regulation. Scientists don't know all the answers yet, but research continues on all these factors and the role they play in development of high blood pressure.

FACTORS CONTRIBUTING TO HIGH BLOOD PRESSURE

THOSE YOU CAN CHANGE	THOSE BEYOND YOUR CONTROL
High Alcohol Intake	Black Race
High Salt Intake	Family History
Inactivity	Increasing Age
Obesity	Male Sex
Oral Contraceptive Use	
Poor Dietary Habits	
Stress	

WHAT CAN I DO TO LOWER MY BLOOD PRESSURE?

To start with, have your blood pressure checked regularly. Ideally, everyone should have his or her blood pressure checked at least once yearly. People with high blood pressure should have their pressure checked more often. Each time you have your blood pressure checked, ask for the numbers. A written record of the date and blood pressure reading will prove very helpful to both you and your doctor in controlling your blood pressure. Since even mild blood pressure elevations increase risk for cardiovascular disease, aim to keep your blood pressure below 120/80 mm Hg.

Follow your doctor's advice. If you are overweight, he or she will probably advise you to lose weight. Blood pressure often drops in direct proportion to weight loss. Many people lose about a point off their systolic pressure (upper number) with every pound of weight lost. Getting rid of excess fat will lessen the work load on your heart and help you look and feel better. Losing weight isn't always easy, but losing even a few pounds can help.

Exercising regularly also helps lower blood pressure by improving circulation and strengthening the heart. In addition, exercise aids in weight control and increases your energy level. Try to exercise fairly vigorously and continuously at least three times a week for 20 minutes or more.

A constant high level of stress may raise blood pressure in some people. Emotions like excitement or anger cause the small blood vessels to tighten, forcing the heart to work harder. Regular exercise helps relieve stress. Also try to set aside time each day for a relaxing activity you enjoy.

The same heart-healthy nutrition plan that lowers blood fat levels helps lower blood pressure. In our practice, we find high-fiber eating lowers blood pressure about 10 percent.

People with high blood pressure will also want to watch their salt intake. Some individuals react to excess salt intake by retaining fluid, putting an extra burden on the heart. Since Americans get about 20 times more salt than they need, it's probably smart for all of us to eat less salt.

To reduce your salt intake, try to stop using salt at the table and cut the amount used in cooking by one-half. Avoid obviously salty processed foods such as potato chips, pretzels, pickles, salted crackers, salted nuts, cured meats, canned soups and stews, and packaged seasoning mixes. Also look for hidden salt in foods disguised as onion salt, garlic salt, monosodium glutamate, or other food additives containing the word sodium.

Some individuals may also need medication to help lower their blood pressure. Currently-used blood pressure medicines include diuretics, "beta blockers" and similar medicines, calcium channel antagonists, vasodilators, enzyme inhibitors, and others. Diuretics help the body get rid of excess fluids and salt. Beta blockers and similar medicines alter nervous system regulation of blood flow through the small blood vessels. Your doctor will decide which blood pressure medicine is the best for you and discuss any side effects.

If your doctor prescribes blood pressure medication, take it regularly. Medication can enhance the blood-pressure-lowering effects of sound nutrition and lifestyle habits, but should not replace these habits. Control of body weight; regular exercise; low-fat, high-carbohydrate and high-fiber eating; and effective stress management will not only help lower blood pressure, but also improve overall health and well-being.

SALT LOWERING TIPS

- Remove the salt shaker from the table.

- Plug half of the holes in your salt shaker by taping over them from the inside.

- Taste your food before salting.

- Cut the amount of salt used in cooking by half.

- Use spices and herbs to enhance the flavor of foods.

- Try some of the reduced salt items.

- Limit foods with soda or sodium listed as one of the first ingredients.

- Limit your use of high sodium seasonings such as steak sauce, ketchup, monosodium glutamate (MSG), soy sauce, garlic salt and onion salt.

- Limit the use of salty foods such as many prepared dinners, canned soups, canned vegetables, cured meats, pickles and salty snacks.

MEDICATIONS THAT HELP LOWER BLOOD PRESSURE

THIAZIDE DIURETICS

(Aquatensen, Diucardin, Diuril, Enduron, Esidrix, Exna,
Hydrodiuril, Hydromox, Hygroton, Lozol, Metahydrin, Naqua,
Naturetin, Oretic, Renese, Saluron, Zaroxolyn)

Action: increases kidney's excretion of sodium and water.
Possible Side Effects: potassium depletion, high uric acid levels.

LOOP DIURETICS

(Edecrin, Lasix)

Action: increases kidney's excretion of sodium and water.
Possible Side Effects: potassium depletion, high uric acid levels,
dehydration, low blood pressure.

POTASSIUM SPARING DIURETICS

(Aldactone, Dyrenium, Midamor)

Action: increases sodium excretion in kidney while sparing
potassium.
Possible Side Effects: high blood potassium.

CENTRALLY ACTING AGENTS

(Aldomet, Catapres, Wytensin)

Action: interferes with stimulation to blood vessels, causing
reduced peripheral vascular resistance.
Possible Side Effects: drowsiness, dryness of mouth, constipation.

BETA BLOCKERS

(Blocadren, Corgard, Inderal, Lopressor, Sectral, Tenormin, Visken)

Action: slows heart rate, reduces cardiac output.

Possible Side Effects: fatigue, sleep disturbances, increased uric acid levels.

VASODILATORS

Apresoline, Loniten

Action: relaxes artery walls.

Possible Side Effects: headache, rapid heartbeat, fluid retention.

ACE INHIBITORS

Capoten, Sarenin

Action: block formation of angiotensin II, a potent increasor of blood pressure.

Possible Side Effects: taste loss, skin rash, headaches.

CALCIUM CHANNEL BLOCKERS

Calan, Cardizem, Isoptin, Procardia

Action: cause dilation of blood vessels and drop in blood pressure.

Possible Side Effects: headache, dizziness, low blood pressure.

ALPHA BLOCKERS

Minipress

Action: dilates some blood vessels, interferes with action of stress hormones.

Possible Side Effects: weakness, dryness of mouth.

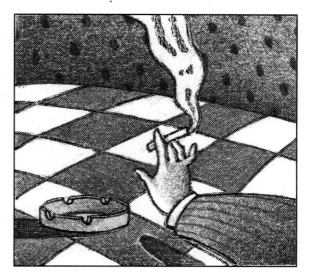

4

SMOKE SIGNALS

One-quarter of all deaths from heart disease relate to smoking, and two-thirds of all smokers die from heart and blood vessel diseases. Cigarette smoking greatly increases your risk for all forms of cardiovascular disease; the more you smoke, the greater your risk. The risk multiplies if you also have high blood fat levels or high blood pressure. Risk is greater for women who smoke and use oral contraceptives, especially for women over age 35.

Even mild smokers run a greater risk of heart and blood vessel diseases. The average smoker smokes one-half pack of cigarettes daily and has three times the risk of stroke compared to non-smokers. The average smoker has twice the risk of heart attack as a non-smoker, and the attack is more likely to be fatal.

Sudden cardiac death occurs two to four times more frequently in smokers than non-smokers. Smoking is also a main risk factor for peripheral vascular disease, a condition where blood flow to the arms and legs is reduced, increasing risk of gangrene or amputation.

Besides cardiovascular diseases, smoking greatly contributes to other diseases. Mild smokers develop lung cancer seven times more frequently than non-smokers; moderate smokers, 12 times more frequently; and heavy smokers, 24 times more frequently. Smokers develop chronic lung diseases like emphysema and chronic bronchitis six to 15 times more frequently than non-smokers. Smoking also increases risk of other cancers, such as cancer of the mouth, larynx, bladder and pancreas.

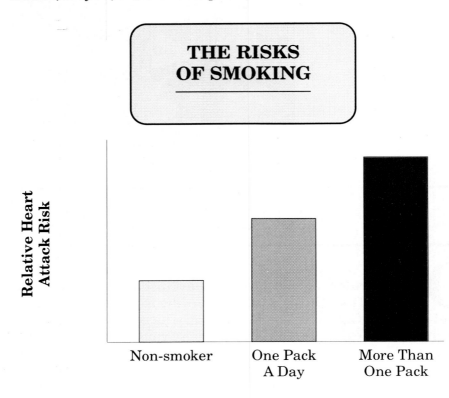

In total, smoking accounts for over 300,000 deaths in the United States yearly. A U.S. government report calls cigarette smoking the "largest preventable cause of death in America." Though the percentage of Americans who smoke cigarettes has dropped in recent years for all groups except teenage girls, over 54 million Americans still smoke. Currently about 35 percent of all men and 28 percent of all women smoke.

HOW SMOKING AFFECTS THE BODY

Cigarette smoke contains many harmful substances. Nicotine is chemically as deadly as cyanide. A single dose of 60 milligrams of nicotine will kill the average adult by paralyzing breathing. The tiny doses of nicotine in cigarette smoke are not enough to kill quickly, but kill gradually by increasing blood pressure, accelerating heart rate by almost 50 percent, and decreasing blood flow to the arms and legs. As the heart works harder, it requires more oxygen.

To make matters worse, another chemical in cigarette smoke called carbon monoxide robs the blood of oxygen and decreases the body's ability to use available oxygen. Angina, or chest pain, can occur because the heart is not getting enough oxygen. In addition, cigarette smoke increases stickiness of platelets in the blood, promoting hardening of the arteries and clot formation.

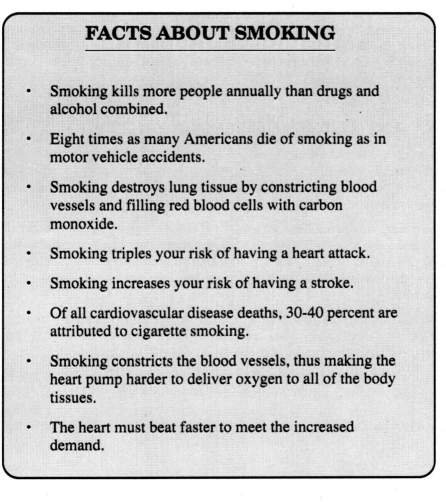

FACTS ABOUT SMOKING

- Smoking kills more people annually than drugs and alcohol combined.

- Eight times as many Americans die of smoking as in motor vehicle accidents.

- Smoking destroys lung tissue by constricting blood vessels and filling red blood cells with carbon monoxide.

- Smoking triples your risk of having a heart attack.

- Smoking increases your risk of having a stroke.

- Of all cardiovascular disease deaths, 30-40 percent are attributed to cigarette smoking.

- Smoking constricts the blood vessels, thus making the heart pump harder to deliver oxygen to all of the body tissues.

- The heart must beat faster to meet the increased demand.

Lung disease can put an additional strain on the heart. Cigarette smoke contains over 4,000 tarry substances that damage lung tissue and promote cancer. Cigarette smoke kills living tissues wherever it contacts them.

EFFECTS ON OTHERS

Smokers aren't the only ones affected by cigarette smoke. Spouses of heavy smokers experience two to three times more lung cancer than people living in more smoke-free environments. Babies born to smoking mothers suffer more complications, birth defects, and low birth weight than babies of non-smoking mothers. Children exposed to smoke in the home get more coughs, colds and ear infections than children of non-smokers.

Since the smoking habit often starts in the teenage years, parents need to set a good example for their children by not smoking. Studies show that if a parent or older sibling smokes, children are much more likely to take up smoking. The smoking habit is much easier to avoid than to break.

ARE ANY FORMS OF TOBACCO SAFE ?

No cigarettes are safe. Using filter cigarettes may not necessarily decrease risk of heart disease because smokers tend to alter their smoking habits to get the same amount of nicotine. They also get more carbon monoxide.

Low-tar and nicotine brands of cigarettes may not offer the promised health advantages either because they contain other cancer-causing substances. Some brands also produce low levels of tar and nicotine in a smoking machine but not when smoked by a human.

Pipes and cigars are also a health risk. Even though the smoke is not as directly inhaled, pipe and cigar smoke is more readily absorbed into the blood stream than cigarette smoke.

Chewing tobacco and snuff are not safe either. Both increase risk of cancer of the mouth and larynx — people who chew snuff have 50 times more cancer of the cheek and gum. People also become addicted to the nicotine and may be more likely to take up smoking.

HOW TO QUIT

Nicotine is one of the most addictive chemicals known to man. Quitting usually isn't easy, but it's well worth it. Immediately after you stop smoking your risk for heart and blood vessel diseases starts falling. Your risk is much lower one to two years after quitting, and about the same as a lifetime non-smoker 10 years after quitting — no matter how many cigarettes you used to smoke daily.

Quitting may take several attempts for some people, but keep trying. Remember the alternatives — stroke, heart attack, lung cancer and other diseases. Some people find it easiest to quit cold turkey; others like to cut down gradually.

You will probably be better able to quit smoking if you first understand your reasons for smoking. Try keeping a smoking diary for a few days, recording when you smoke each cigarette, why you smoked that particular cigarette, and how you felt at the time.

DAILY SMOKING DIARY

Time	# Smoked	Why I "Lit Up"	How I Felt	Situation

Some people smoke to get a lift. If this is you, be sure to get enough sleep and use a substitute activity to perk you up. Exercise is a great pick-me-up. Besides regular exercise lasting 20 to 30 minutes, you can stretch and do a few quick exercises when you would have lit up a cigarette. Try taking a few flights of stairs, a walk down the hall, or doing some easy floor exercises. Chewing gum or taking a cold shower may also help.

If you like to smoke because you like fingering and holding something, substitute another object — a paper clip, coin, pencil or pen. If you smoke to relax, substitute something else relaxing. How about a ten minute nap? Read a book, try some deep breathing, work on a hobby — anything else but don't smoke.

Others smoke when they are tense or angry. If this is you, talk to someone instead of lighting up. Use vigorous exercise to help relieve tension. Quitting may also be easier for you during a vacation or at other less stressful times.

If you crave a cigarette, chew gum, drink water, and keep plenty of fresh vegetables handy to munch on. Try putting the craving off another ten minutes and get busy with an activity — the craving usually goes away.

If you smoke out of habit, learn what situations trigger you to smoke. If you usually smoke at the table after meals, leave the table immediately after eating and have another activity planned and waiting. If you smoke in a certain room at home or work, avoid these rooms as much as you can.

All smokers can benefit by making it hard to smoke. The most obvious step is not to keep cigarettes in the house or work place. If you have to run to the store each time you want to smoke, you will be less likely to smoke. If you must keep cigarettes in the house, try putting them away in an inaccessible place, like the top closet shelf. If you want a cigarette you will have to work to get it.

Once you understand why you smoke, make a conscious decision to quit and decide how you're going to do it. Tell your family and friends your intentions and ask for their support. Put your quitting plan in writing and make a list of your personal reasons for quitting, keeping these posted where you see them often.

Don't be discouraged if you slip off your plan — get right back on. Quitting smoking takes more than one try for many people. Many people also experience withdrawal symptoms when they stop smoking, so prepare yourself for these. You may feel sleepy, restless or hungry. Plan ahead how you will handle these feelings.

You won't automatically gain weight when you stop smoking. One-third of people who stop smoking gain weight, one-third stay the same weight, and one-third actually lose weight. If you feel hungry, snack on fresh fruits and vegetables, which are low in calories and high in fiber and nutrition.

TIPS FOR QUITTING SMOKING

- Try making it one hour without a cigarette, then gradually lengthen the time.

- Make yourself smoke standing up. You will be more aware of what you are doing and enjoy smoking less.

- Change to a brand of cigarettes that you don't like.

- Save up the money you would have spent on cigarettes and buy something special with it. Depending on how much you smoke, this can add up to $250-$1000 yearly.

- Buy only one package of cigarettes at a time.

- Let your cigarette butts pile up in the ashtrays, or better yet, put them in a jar of water and smell the jar every time you think about smoking.

- Join a smoking cessation or support group.

- Keep chewing gum on hand.

- Take a cold shower.

- Take a 10 minute nap.

- Ask for help if you need it.

- Check out reading materials on smoking cessation.

If you feel you need help, don't be afraid to ask. Several sources of information, organizations and programs that can help you quit smoking are listed in the Appendix. Local affiliates of the American Lung Association, the American Cancer Society, and the American Heart Association may have additional information on "stop-smoking" classes in your area and may also be able to connect you with other individuals who have stopped smoking. Many area clinics offer stop-smoking classes. Your local newspaper may also advertise such classes. Your family, friends, and doctor can also encourage you. Several suggested reading materials on smoking cessation are also listed in the Appendix.

Reward yourself after you quit smoking. Think of all the time and money you save by not smoking — use it to do something special for yourself. Don't ever be fooled into having "just one" cigarette. Even years after quitting, "just one" can hook you again. You went through all the effort to quit once, you don't want to do it again.

Kicking the smoking habit will help you look and feel better. You'll be surprised at how much energy you have and how much easier physical activity is. Best of all, your risk of deadly diseases such as heart attack, stroke, and cancer will drop drastically.

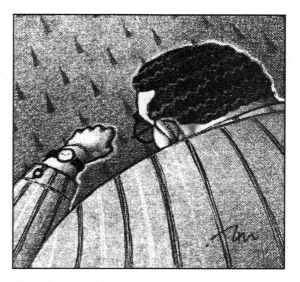

5

WHY WEIGHT?

Excess body fat aggravates many of the risk factors for heart and blood vessel diseases. It also increases risk for heart disease independently and promotes development of other diseases such as cancer of the breast or colon. If you are overweight and have other heart disease risk factors such as high blood pressure, high blood fat levels, or high blood sugar, losing weight is one of the most important steps you can take to lower your risk. For some people, it is the most important step.

Losing weight can be difficult, but losing even 10 to 20 pounds will help reduce heart disease risk. An HCF nutrition plan is ideal for losing weight because of its high fiber and low fat content.

DO YOU NEED TO LOSE WEIGHT?

About 30 to 40 percent of Americans weigh more than they should, including an increasing number of children. Losing weight can help us look and feel our best.

You can get an idea of the body weight right for you by using the quick formula on the following page. The Metropolitan Weight Tables found in the Appendix provide a more extensive listing of desirable weights. Depending on frame size and body build, your desirable body weight might be more or less than listed in those tables.

For some people, a desirable body weight seems hopelessly far away. Try not to be discouraged by this. Setting small, realistic weight loss goals can help you gradually move toward your ultimate weight loss goal. Losing even 10 percent of your current body weight will significantly improve your health. If you weigh 250 pounds, for example, losing 25 pounds will significantly reduce your risk for heart disease, stroke, cancer and diabetes.

HOW MUCH SHOULD YOU WEIGH?

MALES

Allow 106 pounds for the first 5 feet of your height and 6 pounds for each extra inch.

FEMALES

Allow 100 pounds for the first 5 feet of your height and 5 pounds for each extra inch.

EXAMPLES

A male who is 5 feet, eight inches tall should weigh 154 pounds.
5 feet = 106, 8 inches = 48
106 + 48 = 154 pounds Total

A female who is five feet, two inches tall should weigh 110 pounds.
5 feet = 100, 2 inches = 10
100 + 10 = 110 pounds Total

HOW FIBER HELPS

When we first started using diets high in carbohydrate and fiber for diabetes, high blood fats and other conditions, we found some people lost weight without really trying. Often they had trouble eating enough calories to maintain their weight. Spouses reported that they lost weight too.

A high-carbohydrate, high-fiber and low-fat diet promotes weight loss and maintenance for several reasons. Pure carbohydrate and pure protein each provide four calories per gram (a unit of weight). Pure fat provides nine calories per gram, and pure alcohol provides seven calories per gram. Therefore, high-fat foods usually contain over twice the calories per equal weight than high-carbohydrate foods do. If you avoid potatoes, rice, peas, bread, and other high-starch foods because you think these foods are fattening, you are wrong.

You get a greater volume of food for fewer calories when you emphasize carbohydrates and fiber in your diet. Three slices of whole wheat toast with one teaspoon of jelly on each, for example, provide fewer calories than one chocolate eclair. One 10-ounce bag of plain frozen broccoli provides fewer calories than two homemade sugar cookies.

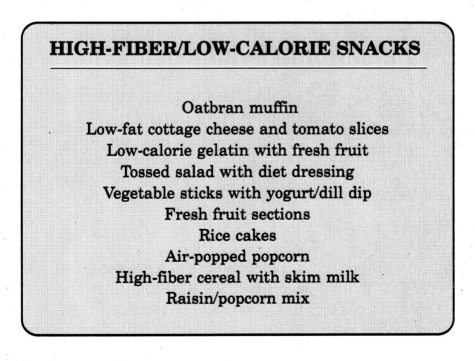

HIGH-FIBER/LOW-CALORIE SNACKS

Oatbran muffin
Low-fat cottage cheese and tomato slices
Low-calorie gelatin with fresh fruit
Tossed salad with diet dressing
Vegetable sticks with yogurt/dill dip
Fresh fruit sections
Rice cakes
Air-popped popcorn
High-fiber cereal with skim milk
Raisin/popcorn mix

High fiber foods are also more filling and satisfying than low-fiber foods. High-fiber foods take longer to eat and tend to stay in the stomach longer. Most of us would feel fuller and more satisfied after eating three small apples compared to drinking the same amount of calories in one cup of apple juice. Some starch is also not as well digested from high-fiber foods as compared to low-fiber foods, so fewer calories get into the body.

CHOOSING THE RIGHT CALORIE LEVEL

Your doctor or dietitian can help you select the right calorie level. You can assist them by first keeping a record of everything you eat and drink for two to three days to determine your current calorie level. The **HCF Lifestyle Record Book** is available through the HCF Nutrition Research Foundation to make this task easy.

Your dietitian can then help you develop an individualized heart-smart eating plan at the right calorie level. To simplify food selection, the dietitian may use a food exchange list, such as those found in **HCF Exchanges**. Instead of counting calories, you just eat the recommended number of servings from each exchange group and you will automatically stay within your calorie limit.

In general, to lose one to two pounds per week you need to cut 500 to 1000 calories daily from your current diet. Mild to moderately overweight women usually lose weight on 1000 to 1200 calories daily. Mild to moderately overweight men usually lose weight on 1200 to 1600 calories daily.

The best way to lose weight is gradually. However, people with large amounts of weight to lose can become discouraged with slow weight loss. If you need to lose more than 70 to 80 pounds or have health conditions that require quick weight loss, you might benefit from a more restricted diet of less than 1000 calories daily. Only your doctor or dietitian should instruct you on such a diet, which usually requires weekly medical supervision.

CALORIE QUIZ

(Answers are on the following page).

1) Which has more calories, a 4 ounce steak or a 4 ounce baked potato?

2) How many calories does it take to make a pound?

3) What food makes a good substitute for sour cream?

4) What are the highest and lowest calorie choices at the salad bar?

5) Which contains more calories, butter or margarine?

6) How many celery sticks could you eat for the same number of calories as one-quarter cup of peanuts?

7) Which is a better fast food choice, a fish sandwich or a grilled cheeseburger?

CALORIE QUIZ ANSWERS

1) Four ounces of grilled sirloin steak contains 317 calories. A 4 ounce baked potato contains only 120 calories. The potato would be more filling, contain less fat and provide more fiber. To fill you up nutritiously, keep meat portions small and plant portions large.

2) About 3,500 calories equals one pound. If you eat just 9 1/2 extra calories per day, you will gain one pound yearly. An extra two packets of sugar in your coffee daily, for example, will add five pounds a year to your weight.

3) Non-fat yogurt! One tablespoon contains only 8 calories, no fat, and tastes almost like sour cream. One tablespoon of sour cream contains 25 calories and 2 grams of fat.

4) High-calorie salad bar choices are high fat ones ... macaroni, potato, chicken and pasta salads made with oil- or mayonnaise-based dressings; cheese and olives; and some of our favorite dressings such as blue cheese, roquefort and ranch. Low calorie choices include the fresh fruits and vegetables such as tomatoes, sweet peppers, hot peppers, carrots, celery, lettuce, onions, and peas. Garbanzo beans are a mid-calorie selection but provide generous amounts of fiber and protein.

5) Butter and margarine both contain 45 calories per teaspoon provided from pure fat! However, butter contains cholesterol and more saturated fat.

6) One-quarter cup of peanuts contains 209 calories. You could eat seven carrots or 10 cups of celery for the same number of calories. Vegetables are more filling and filled with fiber.

7) Fish sandwiches are higher in both calories and fat content than a cheeseburger because they are usually breaded and deep fried. Fish sandwiches with cheese and tartar sauce average 420 calories. A cheeseburger has about 300 calories and a regular hamburger has even less calories and fat.

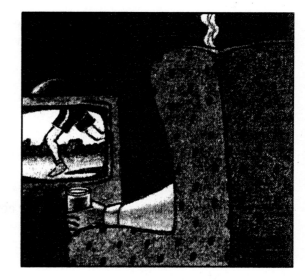

6

KEEP ON MOVING

C huck was a 35-year old slightly overweight finance officer in a large metropolitan bank. He worked intensely at the bank, smoked about a pack of cigarettes daily, and just wanted to relax and watch television when he got home. He never thought of exercising; he felt like he had been active and on his feet all day long.

When his father died of a heart attack at age 63, Chuck decided to quit smoking. In looking for alternative activities over lunch breaks, he and a friend arranged to play tennis a few days weekly. After six weeks Chuck noticed his breathing came easier, his pants were looser, and he had more energy overall.

He began reading exercise information and decided to start a mild jogging program. Chuck started with 20 minutes of mixed jogging and walking over his lunch hour on the days he didn't play tennis. He soon built up to 30 minutes of running three days weekly. Chuck felt more productive at work and had more energy left over in the evenings. Since he watched television less, he snacked less on high-fat foods and also ate a healthier diet.

Marge was 72 years old when she began a healthy eating and exercise program to lower her blood cholesterol level, reduce her blood pressure, and lose weight. She needed to lose about 40 pounds, and had a beginning blood cholesterol level of 263 mg/dl and blood pressure of 160/98 mm Hg.

After a few weeks on a low-calorie, high-fiber diet and after checking with her doctor, Marge began a modest walking program of 10 to 15 minutes four times weekly. She had been active earlier in life, but had not exercised regularly for several years.

Marge soon found she liked to walk and organized some of her neighbor friends to walk with her. After nine weeks on her nutrition program, Marge gradually worked up to walking 30 minutes four days weekly.

Marge lost her 40 pounds in 22 weeks, and her blood cholesterol level and blood pressure returned to normal. She had more energy for other activities and felt more agile. She never knew she could feel so good at age 72.[*]

BENEFITS OF EXERCISE

Regular exercise complements all aspects of heart-healthy eating. It helps lower blood cholesterol and triglyceride levels, raises the protective HDL lipoprotein cholesterol levels, reduces body weight, lowers blood pressure, and promotes a normal blood sugar level.

Exercise strengthens the heart, improves circulation, and helps clear the blood vessels. Exercising regularly is not a guarantee against a heart attack, but it certainly decreases your chances.

Exercise offers many other benefits. It improves your mental outlook and helps most people sleep better. Exercising regularly helps you look better and feel better. It also gives you more energy for other activities.

Regular exercise is good for everyone, but especially for those trying to lose weight. Exercise burns calories and even helps to suppress appetite for some people. When you diet only, some of the weight you lose is muscle tissue. When you combine diet and exercise, you lose less muscle tissue and more body fat.

[*]   *The examples in this book use fictitious names but are based upon actual case studies.*

TYPES OF EXERCISE

Exercise can be grouped into two categories. Aerobic exercises are rhythmical, low-intensity activities you can continue over a longer period of time, such as brisk walking, jogging, swimming, biking, rowing, or cross-country skiing. Anaerobic exercises are those which require a short burst of energy that you cannot keep up very long, such as running a 100-yard dash or lifting weights.

TYPES OF EXERCISE

CONDITIONING AEROBIC	NON-CONDITIONING NON-AEROBIC
Cross-country skiing	Baseball
Cycling	Bowling
Dancing	Croquette
Jogging	Football
Racquetball	Gymnastics
Rope jumping	Horseback riding

Other activities such as bowling, golfing, horse-back riding, tennis, volleyball or yardwork help to burn extra calories but are not usually continuous or intense enough to be aerobic.

Aerobic exercise is the type most beneficial for strengthening the heart and blood vessels, reducing blood pressure, and lowering blood fat levels. You don't need to go overboard with aerobic exercise to achieve the cardiovascular and other health benefits. Try to work up to 20 to 30 minutes of continuous aerobic exercise three or four days weekly. Begin and end each aerobic exercise period with about five minutes of stretching to warm up and cool down. This will help prevent strain or injury to muscles and joints.

The HCF Guide Book tells you how to check your pulse and heart rate to tell if you are exercising too hard or not hard enough. In general, you should be exercising hard enough to make your breathing a little heavy, but not so heavy you cannot carry on a conversation.

GETTING STARTED

If you are over 35 years of age or have a history of heart trouble, check with your doctor before you begin an exercise program. If you have not exercised regularly for a long time, start slowly and build up gradually. Listen to your body — if it hurts or you are stiff and sore the next day, you are probably doing too much too soon. If you experience any of the warning signs listed below, stop exercising immediately and consult your doctor.

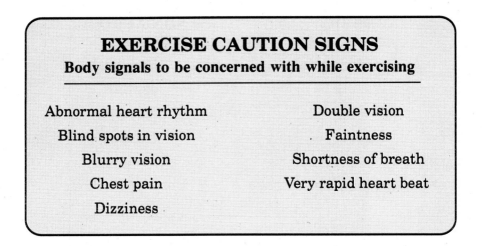

EXERCISE CAUTION SIGNS

Body signals to be concerned with while exercising

Abnormal heart rhythm	Double vision
Blind spots in vision	Faintness
Blurry vision	Shortness of breath
Chest pain	Very rapid heart beat
Dizziness	

Before beginning your exercise program, get the proper equipment to reduce strain or injury to joints and muscles. For most people, this simply means purchasing a good pair of walking or jogging shoes with good arch support and a wide heel base to avoid turning your ankle. Loose, comfortable clothing will also make your exercise time more pleasant.

Choose an exercise you enjoy, or vary your activities if you get bored with one exercise. If you have a physical handicap, an exercise specialist can help develop an exercise program that is right for you. If you decide to join an exercise class, be sure your instructor is well-qualified and that he or she addresses your individual needs.

Almost everyone can start a walking program, even if only to the end of the block and back at first. Walking can be done anywhere, requires no special equipment other than a good pair of shoes, and takes no preparation time other than a warm-up. Just start walking a distance you are comfortable with three to four times weekly and build up at your own pace from there. When you start slowly and build up gradually, you will be surprised how effortless exercise can be.

KEEPING GOING

Choose the type of exercise you think you will enjoy and continue. For many people, the more preparation needed for exercise, the less likely they are to do it. For example, to swim laps at a fitness club you have to get there, change clothes, change back again, and return home. Some days you may not feel like bothering to do this. With walking, jogging, or biking, you just walk out your door and go. However, some people enjoy a more social exercise setting or require a structured exercise class to help motivate them. Plan your exercise time into your schedule, reserving a minimum of 30 minutes of exercise time three days weekly. Many people find it best to exercise right away in the morning. If you wait for free time to exercise later in the day, other things usually come up instead. If your schedule is tight, consider getting up a little earlier, using part of your lunch hour, eliminating something else from your schedule, or combining exercise with another activity, such as riding a stationary bike while you watch the news.

Exercising with someone else can make exercise more enjoyable. Family members can enjoy walking and talking together. Perhaps a neighbor or co-worker would enjoy walking with you. However, if the other person finds excuses to stop exercising, do not let them be your excuse to stop — continue exercising yourself.

Once you have established a regular exercise routine, try not to stop. You lose your endurance much more quickly than it takes to build it up again. If you do stop, get started again as soon as possible. Anticipate busy times when you are likely to stop exercising, such as during holidays or while traveling. Plan ahead how you are going to fit exercise into your schedule on such occasions. Regular exercise is like anything else important in life — you must decide you are going to do it and make time for it. You'll be glad you did.

SAMPLE EXERCISE PLANS

Exercise can be something as simple and easy as a daily walk. When done on a regular basis it can strengthen the heart's ability to work. In addition it can strengthen the bone, relieve some stress and is a safe form of exercise. Choose the plan below that best fits your person. Start each session with a few minutes of stretching exercises and close each session with very slow paced walking. Exercise at least three days per week.

WALKING PLAN A

For the person who has not been exercising and leads a very sedentary life.

WALKING PLAN B

For the person who has been active in his/her daily activities and is in good shape.

WEEK	RATE (mph)	TIME (min.)	WEEK	RATE (mph)	TIME (min.)
1	2.0	10	1	3.5	20
2	2.5	12	2	3.5	20
3	2.5	15	3	3.5	25
4	2.5	17	4	3.5	28
5	3.0	19	5	4.0	30
6	3.0	21	6	4.0	35
7	3.0	23	7	4.0	40
8	3.0	25	8	4.0	45
9	3.5	25	9	4.5	45
10	3.5	27	10	4.5	50
11	3.5	29	11	4.5	55
12	3.5	30	12	5.0	60

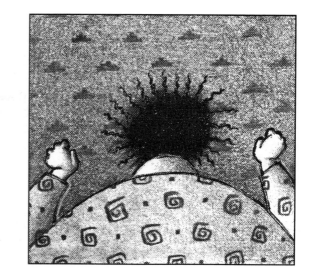

7

PACING YOUR LIFE

Do you often feel frustrated that you don't have enough time? Do you work hard to be at the top in most things you do? Do you let little things get to you? Do you have difficulty just relaxing?

These are some of the traits of the classic "type A" personality pattern, which is characterized by competitiveness, impatience, aggressiveness, time-urgency, and an achievement orientation. For several years experts believed this personality pattern contributed to heart disease. However, recent studies failed to confirm this link.

DOES STRESS CAUSE HEART DISEASE?

The link between stress and heart disease remains tenuous and inconsistent. One recent study even showed people with type A personality recovered better after their first heart attack than more relaxed, easy-going people. Perhaps we are fooling ourselves if we think we can accurately classify personality into broad categories. Or perhaps some other personality characteristic, such as hostility or depression, raises risk for heart disease.

What seems to matter most is the body's own individual reaction to stress. Most of us notice some physical signs of stress, such as clammy hands, dry mouth, or muscle tension.

Certain people may over-react physically to stress, with an out-pouring of adrenalin, increased blood pressure, accelerated heart rate, and heartbeat irregularities. With continual stress over time, these reactions can produce physical harm. Stress can also trigger some people to eat, smoke, or drink too much, which further contributes to heart disease.

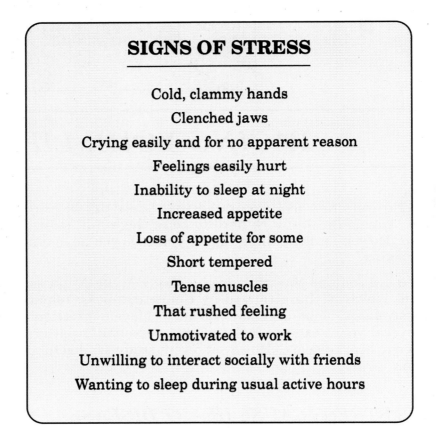

SIGNS OF STRESS

Cold, clammy hands

Clenched jaws

Crying easily and for no apparent reason

Feelings easily hurt

Inability to sleep at night

Increased appetite

Loss of appetite for some

Short tempered

Tense muscles

That rushed feeling

Unmotivated to work

Unwilling to interact socially with friends

Wanting to sleep during usual active hours

THE STRESSES IN YOUR LIFE

Whatever the link between stress and heart disease, most of us enjoy life more when the pace is not so hectic. A certain amount of stress can be good and helps motivate us. Some people even do their best work under stress. But too much stress can wear us down and eventually cause burnout.

Stress is a real part of most of our lives. Major life events, such as marriage, divorce, death of someone close to us, moving, or starting a new job can cause stress.

Often, though, the continual day to day stresses wear at us the most. For many of us, these can include a demanding job schedule, financial problems, strained relationships, noisy children, not enough time, or an endless list of other situations. Some of these situations are under our control; some are not. Try to change stressful situations if you can. If you cannot, perhaps you can change how you think about them.

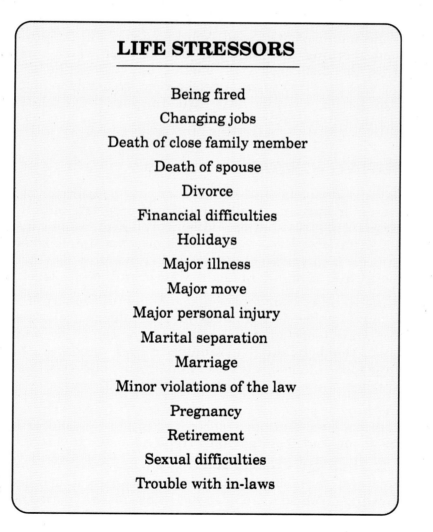

LIFE STRESSORS

Being fired

Changing jobs

Death of close family member

Death of spouse

Divorce

Financial difficulties

Holidays

Major illness

Major move

Major personal injury

Marital separation

Marriage

Minor violations of the law

Pregnancy

Retirement

Sexual difficulties

Trouble with in-laws

People react to the same situation in different ways. In this sense stress is more your perception of a situation rather than the situation itself. Consider the following: You are on a family vacation and your children want to go for a swim in the pool. You are overweight and feel very self conscious in your swimming suit. When you enter the pool area people begin laughing. Someone has just told a joke, but you think they are laughing at you. This situation is very stressful for you because of your perceptions of the situation, which are wrong.

Consider another situation: You left home at the usual time and are on your way to work. You get stuck in a traffic jam caused by an accident a few minutes earlier and have to wait several minutes while policemen clear the road. You know you will be late for an important morning meeting. You look at your watch, tap your fingers on the dash, rev your engine, and watch the progress intently. The situation turns out to be very stressful for you, when instead of fretting you could have turned on your radio, relaxed and enjoyed your extra time.

MANAGING STRESS

When you cannot change a situation or your perceptions of it, the key to stress management is finding the appropriate outlet. Exercise is a natural stress outlet and helps relieve tension caused by stressful situations. Even a short walk or some simple stretching exercises can help you feel better. Regular exercise also increases your energy and stamina, reducing your overall stress level.

Learning to relax your muscles also helps relieve stress. If you notice your forehead is wrinkled, your shoulders are raised and tense, or your teeth hurt because you are clenching your jaw throughout the day, take five minutes to shut your eyes, think of something pleasant, and relax every muscle in your body. Your will feel refreshed and ready to work when you are through.

If something or someone causes you stress, express your feelings instead of bottling them up. Often talking to a friend or family member about your feelings helps tremendously. If you have difficulty talking, write your feelings down.

Take care of yourself by getting adequate rest and relaxation time. Getting involved in hobbies you enjoy such as sports, gardening, crafts, woodworking, or other projects helps take your mind off stressful situations and puts things in perspective.

Different types of outlets work best for different types of people. Find a few outlets that work for you and practice them. For other helpful suggestions you may want to check the resources listed in the Appendix or in the stress bibliography on page five of **The HCF Guide Book.**

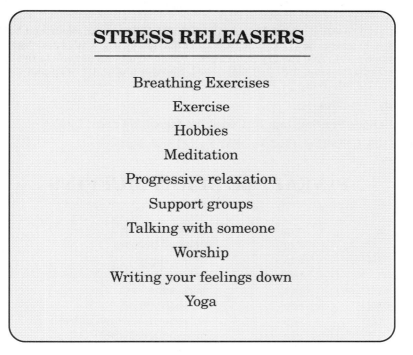

STRESS RELEASERS

Breathing Exercises

Exercise

Hobbies

Meditation

Progressive relaxation

Support groups

Talking with someone

Worship

Writing your feelings down

Yoga

BANANA FRUIT MUFFINS

2	cups	cereal, oat bran
1/2	cup	flour, all purpose
1/2	cup	assorted fruit, dried
1/2		ripe banana
2	teaspoons	baking powder
3/4	cup	milk, skim
1/3	cup	honey
2		egg whites
2	tablespoons	vegetable oil

Heat oven to 400 degrees. In a small bowl mix the oat bran, flour and baking powder. In a large bowl combine the skim milk, honey, egg whites and vegetable oil, mixing well. Add the dry ingredients, the dry fruit and banana to the liquid ingredients, mixing until just moistened. Spray a muffin tin with pan coating and fill 2/3 full. Bake for 17 minutes.

Yield: 12 muffins

Exchanges Per Serving: 1/2 Cereal, 1/4 Starch, 1/4 Fruit, 1/2 Fat

Kcal 139, CHO 22 g., PRO 5 g., FAT 3 g., FIBER 3 g.

PINEAPPLE BERRY MUFFINS

2	cups	cereal, oat bran
1/2	cup	flour, all purpose
1/4	cup	brown sugar
1	tablespoon	baking powder
1/2	cup	milk, skim
1/2	cup	raspberry juice
1/2	cup	strawberries, frozen or fresh
1/2	cup	pineapple, crushed
2		egg whites
2	tablespoons	vegetable oil

Heat oven to 425 degrees. Combine oat bran, flour, brown sugar and baking powder in a small bowl. In a large bowl combine the skim milk, raspberry juice, strawberries, pineapple, egg whites and vegetable oil. Add the dry ingredients, mixing until moistened. Spray a muffin tin with pan coating and fill 2/3 full. Bake for 17 minutes.

Yield: 12 muffins

Exchanges Per Serving: 1/2 Cereal, 1/4 Starch, 1/2 Fruit, 1/2 Fat

Kcal 103, CHO 17 g., PRO 1 g., FAT 3 g., FIBER 3 g.

8

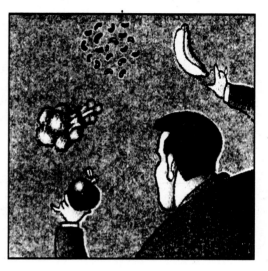

HEART SMART EATING

John was 48 years old and had no history of heart problems when he came to our clinic. He was married and had two teenage children. John ate a typical high-fat American diet, had a blood cholesterol level of 280 mg/dl, and blood triglycerides of 1485 mg/dl.

We started John on a healthy eating plan low in fat and high in carbohydrate and fiber. His whole family adopted the new eating style. After 30 days of healthy eating, John's blood cholesterol fell to 131 mg/dl and his blood triglycerides dropped to 306 mg/dl. He also lost 10 pounds. John significantly reduced his risk for heart and other diseases by making simple changes in the way he was eating. *

We began studying diets high in carbohydrate and fiber and low in fat (HCF diets) for people with diabetes in 1974. We soon discovered these diets also lowered blood fats significantly, promoted weight loss, and decreased blood pressure. I started such

---

* *The examples in this book use fictitious names but are based upon actual case studies.*

a diet myself and lowered my own cholesterol level from 285 to 175 mg/dl.

Since 1974, experience with hundreds of people shows eating the HCF way lowers blood cholesterol levels an average of 20 to 30 percent and blood triglyceride levels 15 to 60 percent, depending on initial levels. HCF eating also lowers blood pressure about 10 percent in people with high blood pressure. Many people on an HCF eating plan lose weight without really trying.

THE HCF EXCHANGE GROUPS

Starches	Beans
Milk	Garden Vegetables
Fruits	Proteins
Cereals	Fats

DIET AND HEART DISEASE

Death rate from heart disease increases as populations eat more animal fat, total fat, animal protein, total protein, calories, meat, eggs, milk, and sugar. Therefore healthy eating is the cornerstone of any program to reduce cardiovascular disease risk. An HCF nutrition plan helps control many of the risk factors for heart disease. HCF eating is healthy, tasty and economical for the entire family.

Following an HCF diet is easy. When you try to change one aspect of your diet, other aspects will automatically change in the right direction. Eating less fat usually means eating less cholesterol and eating more carbohydrate. Adding fiber to your diet increases your carbohydrate intake and lowers your fat intake. Eating the HCF way is really a return to the more wholesome diet our ancestors followed 100 years ago when heart disease was rare.

Your doctor or dietitian can help develop an HCF nutrition plan that is right for you and provide valuable information and encouragement. To begin an HCF eating plan, you will need some tools. **THE HCF GUIDE BOOK** gives a detailed description of the HCF nutrition program, recipes, sample menus, and ideas on following the plan in special situations. **HCF EXCHANGES** lists portion sizes of over 250 foods grouped into eight food categories according to their calorie, protein, fat, carbohydrate and fiber content. Both books will be extremely helpful to you.

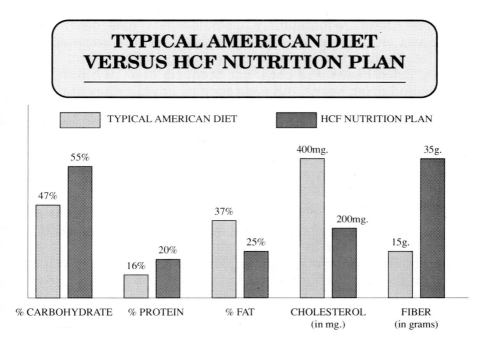

TYPICAL AMERICAN DIET VERSUS HCF NUTRITION PLAN

TYPICAL AMERICAN DIET   HCF NUTRITION PLAN

- % CARBOHYDRATE: 47% / 55%
- % PROTEIN: 16% / 20%
- % FAT: 37% / 25%
- CHOLESTEROL (in mg.): 400mg. / 200mg.
- FIBER (in grams): 15g. / 35g.

FIBER

Many studies show groups of people who eat high-fiber diets have a very low rate of heart disease. The average American male eats about 18 grams of fiber daily, and the average American female, about 13 grams. Many U.S. health organizations now recommend a fiber intake of more than double this amount. Our regular HCF plans provide about 25 grams of fiber per 1000 calories eaten, or about 50 grams of fiber daily.

Fiber is the part of plant foods that is not fully digested in the body. Only plant foods contain fiber — animal foods contain no fiber.

Two main types of fiber exist — insoluble and solublr. Both types seem to help lower blood pressure and promote weight loss, since high-fiber foods usually contain fewer calories than comparable low-fiber foods. Soluble fiber also contributes to satiety and a feeling of fullness by slowing digestion. Insoluble fiber has little effect on blood fat levels. Soluble fiber significantly lowers blood fat levels both by taking fat and cholesterol out of the body and by changing the way the body handles fat.

Insoluble fibers are found more in whole wheat, most other cereal grains, and vegetables, though these foods contain some soluble fiber. Soluble fibers are gummy or gelling-type fibers found more in fruits, dried beans and peas, oat products and psyllium. Oat products and dried beans and peas such as navy, kidney and pinto beans, chickpeas, and lentils are especially rich in soluble fiber. To increase your overall fiber intake, use whole-grain cereal products such as whole-wheat or pumpernickel bread, brown rice, or whole grain breakfast cereals. Also try to eat more fruits and vegetables, leaving the peelings on whenever possible. The peelings are rich in fiber, vitamins and minerals.

To increase your soluble fiber intake, eat more dried beans and peas, oat products, and fruits. We suggest including at least 10 grams of soluble fiber in your diet daily. This means about one-third of the fiber you eat is soluble. The chart below gives average figures on the soluble fiber found in selected food products. Addi-

SOURCES OF SOLUBLE FIBER

1/2	cup	oat bran, dry	=	3.0 grams
3/4	cup	oatmeal, cooked	=	1.4 grams
1/2	cup	cooked beans	=	2.0 grams
1/2	cup	vegetables	=	.8 grams
1	serving	fruit	=	.6 grams
1	slice	whole grain bread	=	.4 grams
1	serving	bran cereal	=	1.2 grams
1	packet	psyllium*	=	2.9 grams

* (Sugar-free Metamucil)

tional information on the fiber content of over 300 foods may be found in **PLANT FIBER IN FOODS.**[*]

As a general rule, including one bowl of oat cereal and two oat bran muffins, one-half to one cup cooked dried beans or peas, or a combination of these foods daily will assure adequate soluble fiber intake. This assumes you use mostly whole-grains and eat at least three servings each of fresh fruits and vegetables daily. Oat cereals include oatmeal, hot oat bran cereal, oat bran flake cereals, or other dry unsweetened oat cereals that list oats or oat bran as one of the first ingredients.

HIGH FIBER CHOICES

CHOOSE	INSTEAD OF
Whole grain bread	White bread
Oatmeal	Refined cereals
Oat bran muffins	Blueberry muffins
Fresh fruit	Fruit juice
Kidney bean chili	Hamburger
Fresh vegetable salad	Cottage cheese with mayonnaise
Vegetable soup	Cream-of-mushroom soup
Fresh fruit cup	Fruit flavored sorbet
Brown rice	White rice
Baked potato with the skin	Mashed potatoes
Stir-fry vegetables	Sweet and sour pork
Whole wheat pasta	Refined pasta

[*] *A complete list of publications available from the HCF Foundation is at the end of this book.*

CARBOHYDRATES

High-carbohydrate foods are those high in starch or sugar. We recommend increasing intake of starch and natural sugars and limiting intake of refined sugars. Foods high in refined sugars usually contain many calories but few vitamins and minerals.

In the HCF exchange lists, the "starches," "beans," and "cereal" exchange groups are the best sources of starch. Garden vegetables also provide carbohydrate. Fruits contain natural sugars but also provide fiber, vitamins and minerals. Foods high in refined sugars include cakes, cookies and candy. Some of these foods also contain large amounts of fat.

The regular HCF nutrition plan includes about 55 percent of calories from carbohydrate, mostly from starch and natural sugars. An aggressive HCF plan might include an even higher percentage of calories as carbohydrate. The average American now gets about 47 percent of his/her daily calories from carbohydrate.

By eating more whole-grains, fruits, vegetables, and dried beans and peas to increase your fiber intake, you will automatically increase your carbohydrate intake. And foods high in carbohydrate and fiber are almost always low in fat and cholesterol. They are also a good source of plant protein, vitamins and minerals.

PROTEIN

The average American gets more than enough protein. Protein is found in animal products such as meat, fish, poultry, and milk; but also in plant products such as grains, dried beans and peas, nuts and seeds.

Many animal protein foods are high in fat and cholesterol. For example, a cooked six-ounce T-bone steak contains 377 calories from fat, or 68 percent of its total calories from fat. In contrast, six ounces of broiled cod contain 178 calories total, only about five percent of which come from fat. Plant protein foods are usually low in fat, contain no cholesterol, and provide generous amounts of carbohydrate and fiber. Nuts and seeds contain more fat than grains, beans or peas, so use them sparingly.

Too often the entire meal revolves around the meat dish. Try to place less emphasis on meat by mixing it with vegetables and grains in casseroles, soups and stews. Try to place more emphasis on other dishes at mealtimes, such as a lightly-seasoned steamed vegetable dish or fresh baked bread.

Use smaller portions of meat. A three to four ounce serving is more than adequate to meet your protein requirements without adding excess fat and calories. Choose the leanest cuts of meat and remove skin or trim visible fat before cooking. Broil, bake or boil rather than fry to reduce fat content. If you do fry, use a non-stick pan or a thin coating of vegetable oil spray.

Try to limit serving red meat to three to four times weekly. Also try to include a few major meatless meals weekly using grains, dried beans and peas, or nuts and seeds.

FAT

Americans eat more fat than people in most other countries. In fact, the average American eats the equivalent of a stick of butter daily.

According to U.S. Department of Agriculture data, Americans get about 37 percent of their calories from fat. Fat in the American diet is often hidden in highly-marbled meats, whole dairy products, or high-fat baked goods. Meats, poultry and fish combined contribute the most fat to the American diet, followed in order by milk products and grain products, with pure fats and oils last.

Most health authorities agree Americans must eat less fat. A high fat intake not only contributes to high blood fat levels and heart disease, but also to weight gain, diabetes, high blood pressure, and certain forms of cancer. Most experts advise eating no more than 30 percent of your calories from fat. Our regular HCF nutrition plan provides 25 percent of calories from fat; an aggressive plan includes even less fat.

The amount of fat you eat affects how much cholesterol and triglycerides your body makes. Most importantly, you want to decrease your total fat intake, no matter what type of fat you eat. Even if you use only liquid margarines and other plant oils, if you use too much of them, your blood fat levels increase.

To reduce total fat intake, use leaner cuts of meat in smaller portions, low-fat dairy products, and plain baked goods. Limit use of butter, margarines, oils, gravies and sauces high in fat. Avoid frying or coating with flour or bread crumbs, which absorb fat.

The type of fat you use also affects your blood fat level. Three types of fats are found in food — saturated, monounsaturated and polyunsaturated. These names refer to differences in chemical make-up of the fats.

TRIMMING THE FAT

- Buy meats that show no visible fat or trim the cuts when you get home.

- Skin poultry before cooking.

- Choose skim milk instead of whole milk.

- Choose lowfat cheeses over regular cheeses.

- Choose sherbet or frozen yogurt over ice cream.

- Have a bagel, English muffin or oatbran muffin for breakfast instead of biscuits.

- Order steamed rice instead of fried rice.

- Switch to reduced calorie salad dressings.

- Use skim milk yogurt in place of sour cream.

- Replace high fat beef cuts such as sirloin with a less fatty meat such as round.

- Cook meat and poultry on a rack, allowing fat to drain off.

- Chill broths, soups and sauces until the fat becomes solid and then spoon off.

- Substitute dry beans and peas for hamburgers.

- Stretch meat portions by mixing with grains and vegetables in mixed dishes.

Saturated fats tend to raise blood fat levels, while monounsaturated and polyunsaturated fats tend to lower blood fat levels. With the exception of fish oils, all animal foods contain mostly saturated fat. Plant foods contain mainly monounsaturated or polyunsaturated fats. The exceptions are palm oil, palm kernel oil, coconut oil, and hydrogenated plant fats such as partially hydrogenated soybean oil, which contain more saturated than unsaturated fat. These fats should be avoided.

While limiting total fat intake, try to eat less saturated fat and more monounsaturated and polyunsaturated fat. Use low-fat dairy products, leaner meats, and less meat. Substitute margarine for butter, and be sure to select a soft margarine with liquid vegetable oil such as corn or soybean oil listed as the first ingredient rather than a partially hydrogenated vegetable oil.

Vegetable oil or margarine can also be substituted in recipes calling for lard or solid shortening. Use vegetable oil sprays or non-stick pans instead of bacon grease or butter, and avoid frying whenever possible. Reading food ingredient lists on food labels can also tell you much about the types of fats used in prepared foods.

CHOLESTEROL

We get cholesterol from the foods we eat as well as from the cholesterol our bodies make. The amount of cholesterol we eat affects how much cholesterol our bodies make.

The average American eats about 400 milligrams of cholesterol daily. The American Heart Association recommends that healthy adults eat no more than 300 milligrams of cholesterol daily, and that people with or at risk for heart disease eat even less cholesterol. If you eat more carbohydrate and fiber and eat less fat, you will automatically be eating less cholesterol. Our regular HCF plans provide about 100 to 200 milligrams of cholesterol daily.

As mentioned earlier, cholesterol is only found in animal foods. One large egg yolk contains 275 milligrams of cholesterol, so try to avoid egg yolks and use egg whites or egg substitutes in place of whole eggs.

Organ meats such as liver, kidneys, sweetbreads and brains are also concentrated sources of cholesterol and should be used only occasionally. Three ounces of cooked beef liver, for example, provide about 370 milligrams of cholesterol. Shellfish such as shrimp, crab and lobster are not as high in cholesterol as previously thought. Three ounces of shrimp contain about 125 milligrams of cholesterol; three ounces of lobster contain about 125 milligrams of cholesterol. Because of the very low fat content of shellfish, we recommend them as good protein-food choices. In general, the lower the saturated fat content of a food, the lower the cholesterol content.

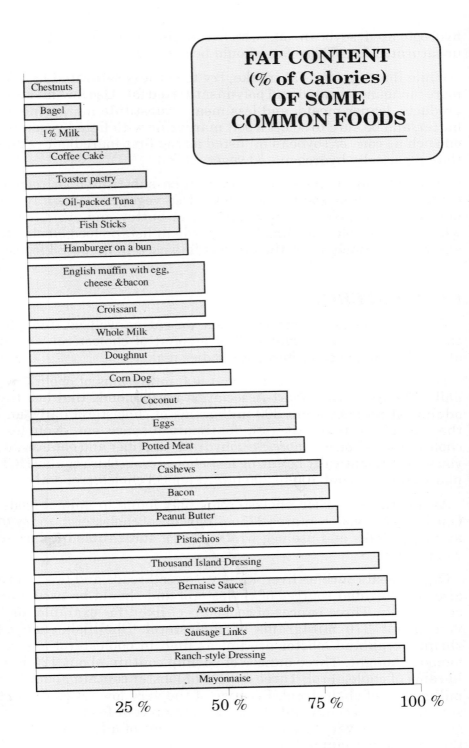

FAT CONTENT (% of Calories) OF SOME COMMON FOODS

Chestnuts
Bagel
1% Milk
Coffee Cake
Toaster pastry
Oil-packed Tuna
Fish Sticks
Hamburger on a bun
English muffin with egg, cheese &bacon
Croissant
Whole Milk
Doughnut
Corn Dog
Coconut
Eggs
Potted Meat
Cashews
Bacon
Peanut Butter
Pistachios
Thousand Island Dressing
Bernaise Sauce
Avocado
Sausage Links
Ranch-style Dressing
Mayonnaise

25 %   50 %   75 %   100 %

SALT

Eating too much salt can raise blood pressure in susceptible individuals. High blood pressure, like high blood cholesterol levels, significantly increases your risk for heart disease and stroke. Even if your blood pressure is normal, it is probably wise not to use too much salt.

The average American eats about 20 times more salt than needed. We would get enough salt even if we never added salt to food and never used prepared foods containing salt.

To cut down on your salt intake, reduce the amount of salt you use in cooking and at the table by one-half or more. Limit obviously salty foods such as potato chips, pretzels, salted crackers, salted nuts and pickles. Also avoid highly-processed and convenience foods such as one-step dinners, packaged seasoning mixes, canned soups and stews, and baking mixes. A few months after kicking the salt habit, you will like the natural taste of foods and think highly salted foods are too salty.

SUGAR

A high sugar intake by itself does not directly raise blood fat levels, blood pressure, or cause heart disease, but it can contribute to all of these by providing excess calories.. A high sugar intake can also raise blood sugar levels in some individuals, which also contributes to heart disease. High-sugar foods such as cakes or cookies are usually high in calories and low in fiber, vitamins and minerals. They can also be high in fat.

We all enjoy the taste of something sweet occasionally, but try to limit your use of refined sugars. Often we can satisfy our sweet tooth by just a taste of something sweet instead of by eating a large portion. If you want to try a luscious dessert in a restaurant, for example, try splitting one piece between four or five people. Hard candy, sherbet, or angelfood or sponge cake taste sweet but contain very little fat. Also enjoy the natural sweetness of fresh fruits. Artificial sweeteners may be used in moderation to sweeten foods or in cooking. When you do use table sugar, brown sugar, honey, or syrups, use them very sparingly.

ALCOHOL

Some studies suggest having one to two drinks daily reduces risk for heart disease by raising protective HDL cholesterol levels. However, other recent studies cast doubt on this idea. Since alcohol provides no vitamins or minerals and many calories, we recommend limiting alcohol intake to two or less drinks daily, or a maximum of 10 ounces of alcohol weekly.

People with high blood triglyceride levels should avoid alcohol completely at first. Even small amounts of alcohol can raise blood triglyceride levels in some people. Once blood triglyceride levels return to normal with other diet and lifestyle changes, some people can resume using modest amounts of alcohol with no effect on their triglyceride levels.

Regular alcohol use is a poor stress management technique. Some people use alcohol to relax or loosen up; some use it to help cope with difficult situations; some use it as an escape. More effective and healthful ways exist to accomplish all of these.

Sometimes individuals drink alcohol because "everyone else does." However, more and more people are choosing non-alcoholic beverages at parties and other social occasions these days. Even if everyone else drinks, make a more healthful choice for yourself by substituting tomato juice, fruit juice, club soda or mineral water with lemon for alcoholic beverages.

If you are pregnant, you should probably avoid alcohol entirely. Even modest alcohol use during pregnancy can damage the developing fetus and cause permanent birth defects.

PUTTING IT ALL TOGETHER

Eating the HCF way can be tasty and wholesome for the entire family and knowing how to assess the nutritional contents will allow you to be sure that your food choices conform to the guidelines for "heart smart" eating. The sample on the following page shows how to calculate the percentage of calories from the information supplied on the labels of your favorite foods.

Our HCF eating plan closely parallels recommendations of many other health organizations, such as the American Heart Association, the National Cancer Institute, and the U.S. Departments of Agriculture and Health and Human Services. Because of concerns that high fiber intake may effect nutrient absorption, we recommend a vitamin and mineral supplement for anyone following an HCF diet.

CALCULATING NUTRIENTS IN A FOOD

$$\% \text{ PROTEIN} = \frac{\text{grams of protein x 4 (calories/gram) x 100}}{\text{total calories per serving}}$$

$$\% \text{ CARBOHYDRATE} = \frac{\text{grams of carbohydrate x 4 (calories/gram) x100}}{\text{total calories per serving}}$$

$$\% \text{ FAT} = \frac{\text{grams of fat x 9 (calories/gram) x 100}}{\text{total calories per serving}}$$

NUTRITION INFORMATION PER SERVING
Serving size .... 4 ounces
Servings per container ...2 ¾
Calories 103
Protein .... 1 gram
Total Carbohydrates .... 9 grams
Simple .... 1 gram
Complex .... 8 grams
Fat .... 7 grams

SAMPLE

$$\text{PRO} = \frac{1 \times 4 \times 100}{103} = 4\%$$

$$\text{CHO} = \frac{9 \times 4 \times 100}{103} = 35\%$$

$$\text{FAT} = \frac{7 \times 9 \times 100}{103} = 61\%$$

The HCF nutrition program is based on an eating plan that is low in fat and high in fiber. This plan is centered around eight food groups or "exchange groups". The food groupings are called "exchange groups" because you can use or "exchange" food within the same list when planning meals. This exchangability gives many options for variety and creativity in meal preparation.

Depending on the calorie level that is right for you, you can have a certain amount or serving from each exchange group daily. The table on the following page suggests two menu pattern options for each of four different calorie levels. Additional information can be found in **HCF EXCHANGES.**[*]

Your doctor or dietitian can help you develop an individual HCF nutrition plan right for you based on the HCF exchange system. In general, people trying to reduce their blood fats should eat no more than SIX ounces of meat on the average, two servings of low- or non-fat milk, at least five to six servings of starches or cereals, at least three servings each of fruits and vegetables, and no more than three to five teaspoons of margarine or other plant oils daily. The meal patterns below and the sample menus found in the Appendix can guide you as you begin your HCF nutrition plan.

HCF MEAL PATTERNS

Exchange Group	1200 calories		1500 calories		1800 calories		2000 calories	
Starch	4	4	6	5	7	7	7	9
Garden Vegetables	3	5	4	4	4	4	3	2
Fruits	2	2	2	3	4	4	5	3
Cereals	1	1	1	2	1	1	2	2
Beans	1	1	1	1	1	2	1	2
Milk	2	1	2	1	2	1	2	1
Proteins	3	4	4	5	6	6	7	7
Fats	5	5	7	6	7	8	8	8

Note- If choosing a meal plan with only one milk exchange, be sure to get your calcium from other foods such as sardines, shrimp, spinach, oysters, turnip greens, salmon (canned with bones), tofu, kidney beans, broccoli and okra. Women may also require a calcium supplement.

[*] *A complete list of the publications available from the **HCF Foundation** is found at the end of this book.*

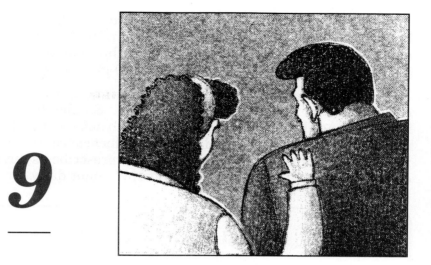

9

WHEN YOU NEED MORE

Perhaps you already have heart disease. Or perhaps you stand a much greater chance of developing heart disease because of a strong family history or other risk factors present. At your doctor's discretion, you may benefit from following a more aggressive HCF nutrition plan.

In contrast to the regular HCF plan, which is healthy for the entire family, the aggressive HCF plan is not for everyone. A physician and registered dietitian must supervise you if you follow this plan, but the potential benefits for individuals with heart disease may be greater than with the regular HCF plan.

Researchers are now studying whether such a diet can stop or even reverse hardening of the arteries.

THE AGGRESSIVE HCF NUTRITION PLAN

The aggressive HCF nutrition plan is a therapeutic prescription for individuals with heart disease and must be monitored by your physician and dietitian. It follows the same principles as the regular HCF plan but takes them further.

The aggressive HCF plan provides more carbohydrate, slightly less protein, and less fat than the regular HCF plan. Of the fat eaten, we pay special attention to getting the right balance of types of fat. Cholesterol intake is limited to 100 milligrams daily.

The aggressive plan also specifies a fiber intake of 70 grams daily, or 35 grams for every 1000 calories eaten. Soluble fiber accounts for about one-third of total fiber intake. To achieve this high fiber intake, you will probably need to use a product concentrated in fiber in addition to eating high-fiber foods. We prescribe psyllium fiber, oat bran and a vitamin and mineral supplement daily.

REGULAR HCF DIET VERSUS AGGRESSIVE HCF DIET

	REGULAR	AGGRESSIVE
Carbohydrate	55%	65-70%
Protein	20%	15%
Fat	25%	15-20% *
Cholesterol	200 mg/day	100 mg/day
Fiber	25 grams/1000 cal.	35 grams/1000 cal. **

* Eat fish twice weekly to increase Omega-3 fats.
** Concentrated soluble fiber is needed. (either one pound dry oat bran weekly or 2 doses of a psyllium product daily).

USING VEGETABLE PROTEINS

When you think of protein foods, you probably think of beef, pork, chicken, fish, and perhaps eggs or milk. These foods are excellent sources of high-quality protein, but they are not the only sources. Grains, nuts, seeds, and dried beans and peas also contain protein. One cup of cooked dried beans, for example, contains as much protein as two to three ounces of meat. To get 65 percent of your calories from carbohydrate and still get adequate protein, you will probably need to make greater use of these vegetable proteins. Vegetable proteins contain no cholesterol, and with the exception of nuts and seeds, they also contain little fat.

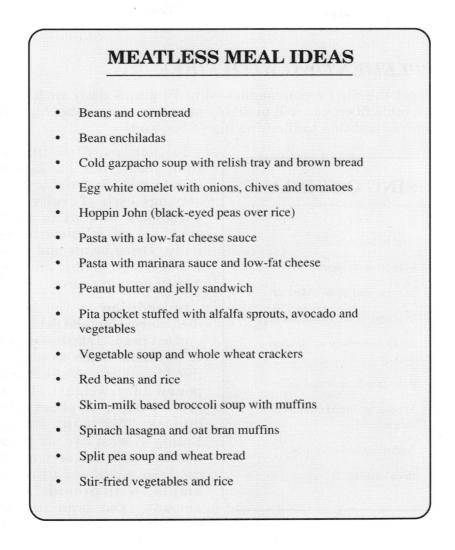

MEATLESS MEAL IDEAS

- Beans and cornbread

- Bean enchiladas

- Cold gazpacho soup with relish tray and brown bread

- Egg white omelet with onions, chives and tomatoes

- Hoppin John (black-eyed peas over rice)

- Pasta with a low-fat cheese sauce

- Pasta with marinara sauce and low-fat cheese

- Peanut butter and jelly sandwich

- Pita pocket stuffed with alfalfa sprouts, avocado and vegetables

- Vegetable soup and whole wheat crackers

- Red beans and rice

- Skim-milk based broccoli soup with muffins

- Spinach lasagna and oat bran muffins

- Split pea soup and wheat bread

- Stir-fried vegetables and rice

You need not become a vegetarian, though this can be a healthy way to eat. You will need to use only small portions of meat and center your diet around vegetables and grains. Try to limit meat servings to two to three ounces at meals, and prepare meatless main meals several times weekly.

Combining vegetable proteins together, or combining a vegetable protein with a small amount of animal protein yields a high-quality protein. Pasta and kidney beans, chickpeas and sesame seeds, peanut butter on crackers, low-fat cheese on bread, or skim milk on cereal are all examples of combinations that yield complete, high-quality protein.

SUPPLEMENTING WITH FIBER

To meet the fiber recommendation of 70 grams daily with one-third soluble fiber, you will probably need to use a product high in psyllium in addition to choosing high-fiber foods.

USING OAT BRAN

- Add to hot cereals

- In muffin recipes

- In meat loaf as an extender

- In soups/stews as a thickener

- As an ingredient in blender shakes

- Bake into breads and rolls

- In place of bread crumbs in recipes

- Add to pancake recipes

- In casseroles

To increase fiber intake from food, your basic diet should include three to four servings each of fruits and vegetables, and six to eight servings of whole grains daily. Dried beans and peas are also high in fiber and are a good protein source.

In addition to the basic diet, we recommend psyllium and oat bran. Take two doses of psyllium such as sugar-free Metamucil. Also eat one pound (dry weight) of oat bran weekly, or about two ounces (2/3 cup) daily. Eating at least two oat bran muffins and one serving of oat bran cereal daily, for example, will provide this amount. Oat bran can be used in the form of hot oat bran cereal or incorporated in muffins, breads, soups, stews and casseroles.

Both oat bran and psyllium are concentrated sources of soluble fiber and lower blood fats significantly. Other types of fiber, such as wheat bran, have little effect on blood fat levels or heart disease risk.

EFFECT OF FATS ON CHOLESTEROL

SATURATED

Action: Raises LDL

Sources: Butter, lard, palm oil or palm kernel oil, hydrogenated shortenings or margarines and coconut oil.

POLYUNSATURATED

Action: Lowers LDL

Sources: Corn oil, cottonseed oil, safflower oil, sunflower oil, soybean oil, fish oil and margarines listing liquid polyunsaturated oil as the first ingredient.

MONOUNSATURATED

Action: Lowers LDL

Sources: Avocado oil, olive oil and canola oil.

MORE ON FATS

To keep total fat intake to 20 percent or less of calories, you will need to use only the leanest meats, limit red meat to two to three times weekly, remove all skin from poultry before cooking, and use small portions. You will also need to choose mostly non-fat dairy products such as skim milk, and use no more than two to four teaspoons of added fat daily.

Added fat should come mainly from plant oils and products using liquid plant oils. Corn, soybean, safflower, sunflower and sesame oils all contain mostly polyunsaturated fat and are good oil choices. Use soft or liquid margarines with these oils listed as the first ingredient.

Avoid palm, palm kernel, and coconut oils, which are more saturated than unsaturated. Also avoid any product with a hydrogenated plant oil listed in the first few ingredients.

New research shows monounsaturated fats also help lower blood fat levels. Populations who eat large quantities of monounsaturated fats such as olive oil have low blood cholesterol levels and low rates of heart disease. Of your added fat, up to one-half of it can come from monounsaturated fats such as olive, avocado or canola oil.

Canola oil is a new type of oil from a plant called rapeseed. It is marketed in the United States under the brand name Puritan oil. Besides being rich in monounsaturated fat, canola oil contains a certain type of fat called Omega-3 fat which also helps lower blood fats.

FISH AND THE OMEGA-3 FATS

New research shows that a special class of polyunsaturated fats called the omega-3 fats significantly lowers blood fat levels. Experimental diets rich in omega-3 fats lower blood cholesterol levels up to 30 percent and blood triglyceride levels up to 60 percent.

Fish are especially good sources of omega-3 fats. It has been known for some time that despite their high fat intake, Eskimos have a very low incidence of cardiovascular disease. Some scientists speculate that this may be a result of the large quantities of fish in their diet.

The higher the fat content of the fish, the higher the omega-3 fat content. Sardines are an especially rich source of omega-3 fats. Salmon, mackerel, haddock, trout and herring are also rich sources. Even though these fish contain more fat than other fish, they are still low in fat and calories compared with other meats.

Because of the low fat and calorie content of fish and because of their omega-3 fat content, we recommend eating fish at least twice weekly. Any type of fish is a good protein-food choice, but you may want to emphasize those fish highest in omega-3 fats. If you use canned fish such as tuna or salmon, be sure to select those packed in water instead of oil. Also be careful not to sabotage your healthy fish choice by adding lots of fat in cooking. Poached, steamed, broiled or grilled fish with lemon is delicious and nutritious.

OMEGA-3 CONTENT
OF SELECTED FISH*

(in a 3.5 oz. serving)

Albacore Tuna .... 1500 mg.

Atlantic Herring .... 1700 mg.

Cod .... 250 mg.

Haddock .... 200 mg.

Halibut, Pacific .... 500 mg.

Mackerel .... 1900 mg.

Oysters .... 500 mg.

Rainbow Trout .... 600 mg.

Salmon, Chinook .... 1500 mg.

Scallops .... 200 mg.

Shrimp .... 300 mg.

Swordfish .... 200 mg.

* From the U.S. Dept. of Agriculture Human Nutrition
Information Service Data Research Branch

PUTTING IT ALL TOGETHER

Your aggressive HCF nutrition plan emphasizes low-fat plant foods and only lean selections of animal foods. A typical aggressive plan will include at least four servings each of fruits and vegetables; six to eight or more servings of whole-grain starches and cereals; a serving of beans; three to four ounces of lean meat, poultry or fish; two servings of non-fat milk; and no more than two to four teaspoons of added fat daily.

In addition, you should use only plant fats for your added fats, mixing monounsaturated and polyunsaturated oil choices. Try to eat fish at least twice weekly, emphasizing those high in omega-3 fats. Also use psyllium and oat bran as concentrated sources of fiber to increase total and soluble fiber intake.

Remember, this type of diet is only for people with or at increased risk for heart disease, and should be started only under the supervision of a doctor and registered dietitian. The meal patterns on the following page and the sample menus in the Appendix can guide you as you begin an aggressive HCF nutrition plan.

AGGRESSIVE HCF MEAL PATTERNS

Exchange Group	1200 calories		1500 calories		1800 calories		2000 calories	
Starch	4	5	5	6	7	8	7	9
Garden Vegetables	2	2	6	5	5	6	5	5
Fruits	4	3	5	4	5	5	6	7
Cereals	1	2	1	1	2	2	2	1
Beans	1	1	1	2	2	1	2	2
Milk	2	1	2	1	2	1	2	1
Proteins	1	2	2	2	2	3	3	4
Fats	5	4	6	6	7	7	8	7

Note- If choosing a meal plan with only one milk exchange, be sure to get your calcium from other foods such as sardines, shrimp, spinach, oysters, turnip greens, salmon (canned with bones), tofu, kidney beans broccoli and okra. Women may also require a calcium supplement.

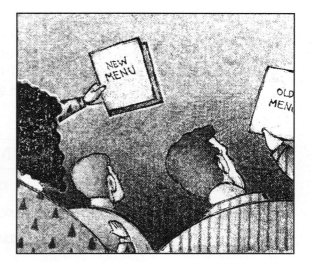

10

MAKING THE CHANGE

Making the change to an HCF nutrition plan is easy if you do it gradually. Once you become familiar with the plan, you won't need to spend any more time in food preparation than you do now. You'll probably save money on your food bill, since foods like dried beans and peas, most cereals, bread, and even fruits and vegetables cost less than traditional high-fat and convenience foods like prime cuts of meat, prepared dinners, or snack foods.

Best of all, you and your family will enjoy better health and well-being on your HCF nutrition plan, since this eating style lowers blood fat levels, reduces blood pressure, helps control blood sugar, and promotes weight loss and maintenance.

PLANNING AHEAD

We are all creatures of habit, and we often eat a certain way because that is what we are used to. When you first adopt an HCF eating style, you'll need to re-think your food selection and preparation. You won't need to give up all your favorite foods or recipes, but you may need to adapt high-fat or high-calorie recipes and limit quantity or frequency of certain foods. Many heart-healthy changes come easily if you plan ahead — and many small changes put together can make a big difference in how healthy your diet is. Switching from whole to low-fat milk, or from low-fat to skim milk, changing brands of margarine, substituting fresh fruit for sweet desserts, choosing a different breakfast cereal, or broiling rather than frying are all examples of changes many people make easily if they plan ahead.

SAMPLE DAILY MENU

	BREAKFAST	LUNCH	DINNER	SNACK
MONDAY	oatmeal raisins skim milk	vegetable soup whole grain crackers fresh apple skim milk	broiled flounder navy beans broccoli salad with oil and vinegar	popcorn oat bran muffin margarine vegetable juice

Other changes might be harder to make, such as reducing serving portions of meats or learning to make meatless dishes. Browse through some new recipe books for ideas or experiment with adapting your own recipes. If you try one new recipe a week, you will soon have a good selection of healthy main dishes. Even if you don't like to cook or don't have the time, you can easily follow an HCF nutrition plan with simple, basic foods. A fresh vegetable salad topped with low-fat cheese, garbanzo beans, and diet dressing and served with rye crackers requires little preparation and makes a very healthy meal. Baked fish with lemon, baked potato, steamed vegetables and whole-wheat toast also takes little creative input but is very healthy.

Many supermarket delicatessens offer healthy food choices such as light salads, steamed vegetables, marinated fish, or sliced turkey or chicken. If you make careful choices, you can even follow an HCF plan while eating mostly at restaurants.

Whether or not you like to cook, try planning your weekly menus on paper ahead of time. You might even plan your snacks ahead. Preplanning reduces impulse eating and allows you to make a more thorough shopping list. You'll probably save time by not wondering what to cook each day and running to the store to get missing ingredients. If the menu is decided ahead, other people might also find it easier to help with food preparation. You can even save the weekly menus for future use.

DOING IT GRADUALLY

Make the change to an HCF nutrition plan gradually. You might first keep a record of everything you eat and drink for three to five days, then study the record. What things are you doing right? What things need changing? Which habits will be easy to change and which will be harder? A registered dietitian can help you analyze your food records and suggest areas for change.

Next, make a list of habits that need changing. Start with the easy ones, then gradually tackle the harder ones, one habit at a time. You might check your progress once or twice monthly by keeping a food diary. Soon the HCF eating style will become habit and heart smart food choices will come automatically.

A FAMILY AFFAIR

The entire family benefits from healthy food choices. Even children can follow a regular HCF nutrition plan, though very young children may need extra fat in their diet for adequate calories. As you adopt the HCF eating style, you invest in your children's future health and teach them healthy habits to last their lifetime.

If necessary, one family member can easily follow an aggressive HCF plan while the rest of the family follows a regular HCF plan by adjusting portion sizes, supplementing with fiber, and occasionally substituting certain foods for other foods.

Though healthy eating is each individual's responsibility, the person or persons in charge of most shopping and cooking duties can help their families make healthy food choices by controlling availability of foods and fixing healthy foods in creative ways.

We want our spouses to lose weight and lower their cholesterol level to live longer, but then we feed them eight ounces of prime rib, fried potatoes and apple pie for supper. We want our children to snack on fresh fruits and vegetables but then we bury these foods behind the soda pop, chocolate cake, potato chips and cheese curls. The best way to help control intake of unhealthy foods is not to buy them or bring them in the house.

IS IT TIME TO MAKE A CHANGE ?

If you:

- have two or more egg yolks weekly

- eat mostly white bread

- eat highly sugared or refined breakfast cereals

- use high fat meats such as bacon, sausage, and hot dogs

- cook or consume butter, lard, coconut or palm kernel oils

- eat fast food meals of burgers, fries and sweet drinks

- choose high fat cheeses such as cheddar, swiss or provolone

- choose salad bar items such as macaroni, potato, pimento cheese and ham salad

- use whole milk

- use gravies, creamed soups, or mayonnaise type dressings

- seldom eat fresh fruits or vegetables

- usually fry foods

- or eat larges portions of meat

Then You Need To Consider Changing To A More Heart Smart Eating Pattern

SPECIAL SITUATIONS

Special situations like eating out, traveling, holidays and vacations provide handy excuses to indulge in fat- and calorie-laden foods. Though an occasional splurge may not hurt and can often be balanced by alternate food choices at home, an HCF eating plan can easily be followed in these situations.

If you eat lunch away from home every day, try bringing your own lunch. Sandwich fillings could include home-cooked or deli turkey or chicken, tuna or salmon, low-fat cheese, mashed beans or a bean spread, or even shredded vegetables and sprouts. Several low-fat cold cuts are available, though most are high in salt. Cottage cheese blended with lemon, mustard, or pickle relish can substitute for butter, margarine or mayonnaise. Dark rye or 100 percent whole wheat bread maximizes fiber content.

For something different, try bringing salads, soups or leftovers. Many work places now have microwave ovens, but a thermos works fine too. Fresh fruits and vegetable sticks round out any brown bag lunch.

When you do eat at restaurants, whether for lunch, while traveling, for convenience or on special occasions, try to choose a restaurant that offers low-fat entrees you like.

Oriental restaurants are often good choices because they serve dishes abounding in rice and vegetables with little meat. Buffets allow you to select individual foods that fit into your meal plan, but don't be tempted to "get your money's worth" by eating everything. Many restaurants offer salads and vegetarian or low-fat entrees. If you look hard enough you can find something healthy to eat at almost every restaurant.

Even fast food restaurants usually have a salad bar, but stick to the plain fruits and vegetables and be careful not to douse your salad with salad dressing or bacon bits. Many people carry their favorite diet dressing in their pocket or purse.

Learn to ask how foods are prepared and make special requests, such as requesting that fish be broiled with lemon rather than fried in fat, that the skin be removed from chicken before cooking, that a salad dressing be served on the side, or that the nacho chips not be brought to the table. You might ask if you can substitute vegetables for the french fries, or order a side dish of vegetables. Remember, you are paying the bill and the restaurant personnel are there to serve you.

Also remember you don't have to eat everything served you just because it is there. Restaurants often serve much larger portions than needed. You might even want to split a meal with someone.

If you travel frequently and tire of eating in restaurants, you might consider taking some food with you. You can usually pack fresh, non-perishable fruit, whole-grain crackers, or cereal. You can even keep a small carton of milk cold in a hotel room ice bucket for a whole-grain cereal breakfast. If you travel by car, such as on a family vacation, you could bring a larger selection of food in a cooler.

Holidays, especially the season between Thanksgiving and the New Year, can test our healthy eating habits. Many traditional holiday foods such as turkey, cranberry salad, popcorn balls, and homemade breads fit into a heart-healthy eating plan. If you serve the meal, you can plan ahead to offer other healthy food choices. If you are invited to someone else's house for a holiday meal, you can offer to bring something. Also try to remember the true spirit of the holidays and focus on the fellowship instead of the food.

Whatever the special situation, you will feel better and do your body a favor if you make healthy eating a priority in your life.

HEART SMART FOOD TIPS

FOR THE HOME

- Use more whole-grain flour and food products.
- Keep oatmeal, oat bran and a variety of beans on hand.
- Use low-fat milk and milk products.
- Include fish in your meals two to three times weekly.
- Choose low-fat red meats, poultry and pork.
- Flavor foods with herbs, spices and wines instead of salt and fat.
- Include complex carbohydrates such as pasta and rice with meals.
- Bake, boil or grill instead of frying foods.
- Serve fresh fruits and vegetables with meals.
- Try some meatless main dishes.
- Use less added fat in recipes and at the table.

EATING OUT

APPETIZERS

- Broth or broth-based soups
- Antipasto (without the high-fat meat and cheeses).
- Hard Rolls
- Fresh Fruit Cup
- Seafood cocktails

SALADS

- Spinach
- Sliced tomatoes and cucumbers
- Oil & vinegar dressing
- Low-fat cottage cheese & tomatoes
- Tossed
- Hearts of palm
- Vinegar-based dressings
- Low-calorie dressings

ENTREES

- Grilled, poached or broiled fish.
- Baked or broiled lean pork or beef.
- Have sauces served "on the side"
- Request that items be prepared in little or no fat.
- Ask for extra vegetables or a vegetable plate.
- Eat less meat.
- Remember, you don't have to eat everything that is served!

BREADS

- Whole grain rolls
- Bran muffins
- Bagels
- French bread

- Hard rolls
- English muffins
- Pita pockets
- Sourdough bread

DESSERTS

- Fresh fruit
- Sherbets
- Angel food cake

- Sorbets
- Sponge cake

- If you want to try a high-fat, high-calorie dessert, one serving can be split between four or five people.

AT THE GROCERY

- Add new fruits and vegetables to your favorite selections.

- Read the labels to learn the fat and fiber content of your favorite foods.

- Search out new low-fat choices in the meat and cheese sections.

- Purchase both dried and canned beans and peas.

- Try some of the many whole-grain products available such as whole wheat pasta, brown rice or whole grain breakfast cereals.

- Choose polyunsaturated oils and margarines.

- Fine a vinegar-based diet salad dressing that you like.

- Purchase ingredients to make foods from scratch rather than purchasing prepared and convenience foods.

- Buy egg substitutes instead of real eggs.

A HEART SMART SHOPPING LIST

- ☐ Bulgur
- ☐ Diet soft drinks
- ☐ Dried beans and peas
- ☐ Egg substitute
- ☐ Extra lean ground beef
- ☐ Fish
- ☐ High fiber cereals
- ☐ Lean luncheon meats
- ☐ Lean meat cuts
- ☐ Low calorie dressings
- ☐ Low fat cheeses
- ☐ Low fat yogurt bars
- ☐ Oatmeal and oat bran
- ☐ Popcorn
- ☐ Poultry
- ☐ Pretzels
- ☐ Sherbet or sorbets
- ☐ Skim milk
- ☐ Skim milk powder
- ☐ Skim milk yogurt
- ☐ Vegetable based soups
- ☐ Vegetable juices
- ☐ Whole grain breads
- ☐ Whole grain crackers
- ☐ Whole wheat pasta

RED BEAN LASAGNA

1	large	onion, chopped
2	medium	carrots, chopped
1	clove	garlic, minced
2	T.	cooking oil
1	16 oz can	tomatoes, cut up
1	16 oz. can	red beans, drained
1	t.	sugar
1/4	cup	parsley, snipped
3	T.	parsley
1	t.	dried oregano, crushed
1	t.	dried basil, crushed
1	t.	salt
10	oz.	frozen spinach, thawed
2	cups	mushrooms, sliced fresh
1		egg substitute
1-1/2	cups (6 oz.)	Mozzarella cheese, shredded
1-1/2	cups	low-fat cottage cheese, drained
1/4	cup	Parmesan cheese, grated
6		lasagna noodles, cooked

Cook onion, carrots, and garlic in oil. Add undrained tomatoes, beans, 1/4 cup parsley, sugar, oregano, basil, and salt. Bring to boiling. Cover; simmer 15 minutes. Mash beans slightly. Add mushrooms, and spinach; simmer, uncovered, 15 minutes. Combine egg substitute, half of mozzarella cheese, the cottage cheese, Parmesan cheese, and 3 tablespoons parsley.

Spread 1/2 cup bean mixture in a 10x6x2 inch dish. Arrange two noodles atop. Spread with one-third of the cheese mixture, then one-third the remaining bean mixture. Repeat the layers twice. Bake, covered in a 375 degree oven for 40 minutes. Top with the remaining cheese. Bake 5 minutes more uncovered.

Yield: 8 servings (1 cup per serving)

Exchanges Per Serving: 2 Protein, 1 Starch, 1 Garden Vegetable, 1 Fat

Kcal 240, CHO 209, PRO 219, FAT 8 g., FIBER 5 g.

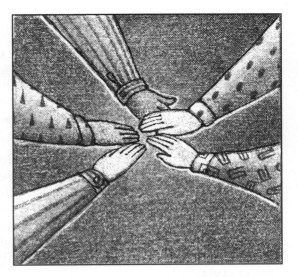

11

YOUR HEART HEALTH TEAM

You are the central player in the challenge to reduce your heart disease risk. You must take the responsibility to identify and change major threats to your health, such as high blood fat levels, high blood pressure, smoking, obesity, inactivity, and poor eating habits. But many people, organizations and materials are available to help and support you as you make these changes.

FAMILY AND FRIENDS

Your family and friends can provide great support and encouragement as you tackle each risk factor for heart disease. They are the ones that care about you the most.

Bring a family member with you to health care appointments and classes. An understanding person can help lend you support. The HCF nutrition and lifestyle plan is healthy for everyone, and your family will also benefit from adopting these new habits. Talk to your family and friends about your diet and lifestyle goals and ask for their help.

HEALTH CARE PROVIDERS

Your doctor coordinates your health care. He or she will order appropriate blood tests, check weight and blood pressure, review lifestyle habits, recommend areas for change, prescribe any necessary medications, help you formulate an overall treatment plan, and provide on-going follow-up. He or she can also identify other health problems.

The doctor may refer you to other health care providers with special areas of expertise. A registered dietitian, for example, provides detailed information on diet and food choices. He or she can assess your current eating habits and help you develop a personal HCF nutrition plan based on your food likes and dislikes. The dietitian can see you on a regular basis to provide support and answer questions as you and your family gradually adopt an HCF eating style.

A nurse or health educator might be particularly helpful in answering day-to-day questions on heart disease, stroke, or use of medications. They might also direct you to written materials or classes in your area.

Schedule regular health care visits and keep the appointments. Make a list of symptoms, questions or concerns to discuss with your doctor or health care provider. Ask for specifics, and keep a record of blood pressure, blood fat levels, body weight, or other pertinent information for future appointments. At a minimum, everyone over 40 years old should have a yearly physical. If you have heart disease or threatening risk factors, your doctor may want to see you more often than this.

YOUR HEALTH CARE TEAM

There are other members of a health care team you may meet with occasionally depending on your individual needs. There are others who are part of your support system that you can turn to when needed.

ORGANIZATIONS

Several organizations can help you manage heart disease risk factors. These organizations often have local affiliates that sponsor health fairs, seminars or classes in communities. They can also offer support and provide a wealth of printed literature. For more information, call or write the individual organization of interest.

READING MATERIALS

Many books and publications can provide fresh ideas and encouragement in specific areas. Not all health and nutrition books are credible, so be careful what you read. Stop at your local library or bookstore for recommended reading materials in the areas that interest you.

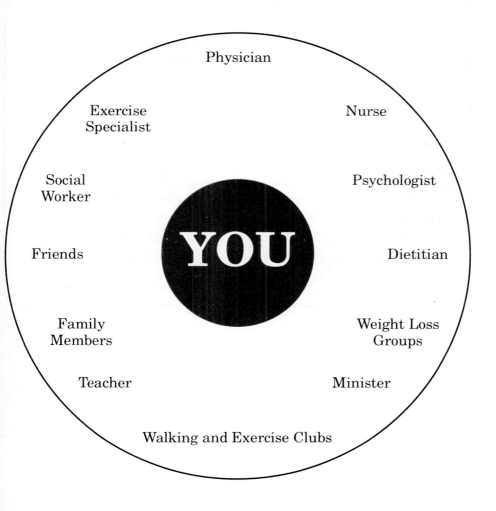

VEGETARIAN SANDWICH

1	cup	cucumber, thinly sliced (unpeeled)
1/2	cup	carrot, grated
1/4	cup	green onions, sliced
3	T.	Italian salad dressing, low-calorie
1	T.	cream cheese, light
2	slices	bread, whole wheat
1/2	cup	alfalfa sprouts
as		

Combine cucumber, carrot, green onions and the Italian salad dressing, toss gently and set aside. Spread the cream cheese over the bread. Spoon the vegetable mixture over the cheese. Garnish with alfalfa sprouts.

Yield: 1 sandwich

Exchanges Per Serving: 3-1/2 Garden Vegetables, 2 Starches, 1 Fat

Kcal 310, CHO 69.5 g., PRO 10.5 g., FAT 47 g., FIBER 11 g.

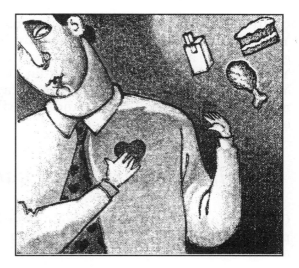

12

PUTTING YOUR HEART IN IT

A bout seventy-five percent of all heart disease and strokes are preventable through diet, exercise and lifestyle changes. Humans are creatures of habit. Take a little time now to change some of your not-so-healthy habits; you will probably live longer and enjoy life more because of the changes.

A diet low in fat and cholesterol and high in complex carbohydrates and fiber, regular exercise, maintenance of a healthy body weight, stress management, non-smoking, regular health care visits, and medications if necessary will all greatly lessen your risk of developing cardiovascular disease.

Changing lifelong habits such as food intake or exercise patterns may take some determination and preplanning at first. Make a list of the changes you need to make, prioritize them, then work on them one at a time. Confront any excuses that keep you from making the changes you need to make. You can keep track of your progress using a lifestyle record book such as the one published by the HCF Foundation.

After a short time, the changes you have made will come easily. You will automatically buy whole grain bread or brown rice at the grocery store and fix your favorite high-fiber recipes from memory. You will think whole milk and high-fat dishes taste much too heavy. You will look forward to your exercise and relaxation times, and miss them if you skip them. And you will look better, feel better, and probably live longer.

The time to start these changes is now...

Consider the alternatives. Your family, friends, health care providers, and several organizations can provide much support and advice.

...but in the end its up to you!

BE HEART SMART GOALS

GOOD

- Blood cholesterol less than 200 mg/dl.

- HDL cholesterol over 45 mg/dl for men and over 58 mg/dl for women.

- Blood triglycerides less than 250 mg/dl.

- Blood pressure less than 140/85 mm Hg.

- Body weight within 10 percent of desirable weight.

- Walk 12 miles weekly or do other aerobic exercise lasting 20 minutes at least three times weekly.

BEST

- Blood cholesterol less than 150 mg/dl plus your age, or less than 200 mg/dl.

- HDL cholesterol over 52 mg/dl for men and 68 mg/dl for women.

- Blood triglycerides less than 150 mg/dl.

- Blood pressure less than 120/80 mm Hg.

- Body weight at desirable level.

- Walk 20 miles weekly or add eight miles walking to other aerobic exercises.

SHARED GOALS

- Non-smoking.

- No more than two alcoholic beverages daily, or 10 ounces of alcohol weekly.

- Effective stress management.

- Regular health care visits.

- High-carbohydrate, high-fiber, low-fat eating style.

GLOSSARY

Aerobic Exercise: Rhythmical, repetitive exercise which increase heart rate and promotes cardiovascular fitness. Examples include brisk walking, jogging, swimming or biking.

Anerobic Exercise: Exercise which requires short, intense burst of energy and builds muscle strength but does little to promote cardiovascular fitness. Examples include sprinting, weight lifting o isometrics.

Angina: Recurring, dull chest pain caused by inadequate bloo supply to the heart.

Arteriosclerosis: A hardening and thickening of blood vessels tha carry blood from the heart to body tissues. A variety of conditions ca cause arteriosclerosis, which is also called hardening of the arterie

Artery: A blood vessel that carries blood from the heart to bod tissues.

Atherosclerosis: Hardening of the arteries caused by build up c cholesterol and other fatty materials in the inner layers of the arter walls.

Blood pressure: The force of blood pushing against the artery wall

Calorie: A unit of energy used to measure both energy value of food and energy value of physical activity.

Carbohydrate: One of three calorie-yielding nutrients concentrate in foods like grains, cereals, fruits and vegetables. Pure carbohydrat supplies four calories per gram.

Carbon monoxide: A chemical in cigarette smoke that deprives th body of oxygen and promotes hardening of the arteries.

Cardiovascular Disease: Diseases involving the heart or bloo vessels.

Cerebrovascular Accident: A stroke

Cholesterol: A waxy, fat-like substance found only in animal tissu that is essential for certain bodily functions. Too much cholesterol i the blood promotes hardening of the arteries.

Complex Carbohydrate: A desirable type of carbohydrate tha includes starches and dietary fiber. Foods rich in complex car bohydrate include breads, rice, pasta, cereals and starchy vegetable

Congestive Heart Failure: A condition where the heart is weakened and cannot pump blood efficiently, often causing fluid to build up in the ankles, legs, lungs and other tissues.

Coronary Artery Disease: Hardening of the arteries feeding the heart, reducing blood flow to the heart muscle.

Diabetes: A metabolic condition where the body does not metabolize nutrients normally because of inadequate production or use of a hormone called insulin. High blood glucose levels are a key sign of diabetes.

Diastolic blood pressure: The lower number of a blood pressure reading, representing the force of blood against blood vessel walls between heartbeats.

Fat: One of three calorie-yielding nutrients in foods, concentrated in foods like butter, margarine, oils, certain meats and regular dairy products. Pure fat provides nine calories per gram—over twice the calories pure carbohydrate or pure protein provides per gram.

Fiber: A variety of substances which are not broken down by enzymes in the small intestine. Fiber is found only in plant foods.

HCF exchanges: A system of grouping foods into eight categories based on similar calorie and nutrient content. The HCF exchange groups emphasize foods high in carbohydrate and fiber.

HCF nutrition plan: A healthy way of eating that is high in carbohydrate and fiber and low in fat.

Heart attack: Death of or damage to part of the heart muscle caused by inadequate blood supply to the heart.

High blood pressure: A condition where the heart must work harder to pump blood through blood vessels. High blood pressure is usually defined as a blood pressure reading of 140/90 mm Hg or more.

High-density lipoprotein(HDL): A good type of lipoprotein that contains mostly protein and helps rid the body of excess cholesterol.

Hydrogenation: A chemical process whereby hydrogen atoms are added back to unsaturated fats, making them more saturated. Hydrogenation improves shelf life but makes a fat more damaging to the heart and blood vessels.

Hyperlipidemia: High blood fat levels, usually referring to high blood cholesterol or triglyceride levels.

Hypertension: High blood pressure.

Insoluble fiber: A type of fiber that helps relieve constipation but does little to lower blood fat levels. Wheat, most other cereal grains, and vegetables contain primarily insoluble fiber

Lipoprotein: Substances made up of fat (lipid) and protein that transport fat and cholesterol in the blood.

Low-density lipoprotein (LDL): A bad type of lipoprotein that contains mostly fat and cholesterol. Low-density lipoprotein is particularly prone to clog blood vessels and contribute to heart disease or stroke.

Monounsaturated fat: A type of fat that contains one double bond in its chemical make-up and helps lower blood cholesterol levels. Monounsaturated fats come mostly from plant foods and include olive and canola oil.

Myocardial infarction: A heart attack.

Nicotine: A toxic product in cigarette smoke.

Oat bran: The outer coating of the oat kernel richest in fiber content. Oat bran is an especially good source of soluble fiber, the kind of fiber that lowers blood cholesterol levels.

Obesity: A condition where body weight exceeds 20% of desirable body weight due to excess fat stores. Obesity increases risk for many diseases, including heart disease, diabetes, and certain cancers.

Omega-3 fat: A type of polyunsaturated fat found in fish oils. Omega-3 fats help lower blood fat levels, particularly triglyceride levels.

Platelets: Sticky cells in the blood that help with normal blood clotting but may also play a role in hardening of the arteries and dangerous blood clot formation.

Polyunsaturated fat: A type of fat that contains many double bonds in its chemical make-up and helps lower blood cholesterol levels. Polyunsaturated fats are usually liquid vegetable oils such as corn, cottonseed, safflower, sesame seed, soybean, or sunflower oils.

Progressive relaxation: A system of progressively relaxing each muscle in the body until the whole body is relaxed and free from tension.

Protein: One of three calorie-yielding nutrients in foods and needed to build and repair muscle, bone, skin and blood. Pure protein provides four calories per gram and is found in milk, cheese, meat, fish, poultry, dried beans and peas, nuts and seeds, and grain products.

Psyllium: A plant derivative used in some laxatives which is a concentrated source of soluble fiber and helps lower blood cholesterol levels.

Saturated fat: A type of fat that contains no double bonds in its chemical make-up and that raises blood cholesterol levels. Saturated fats are usually solid at room temperature and come mostly from animal foods like butter, lard, high-fat dairy products, and fatty meats. A few vegetable foods like coconut, palm, and palm kernel oils also contain mostly saturated fat.

Simple carbohydrate: A type of carbohydrate that includes natural sugars from fruits, milk, honey or grains; and refined sugars from table sugar, candy, cakes, cookies and pies.

Soluble fiber: A type of fiber that helps lower blood fat levels. Oat bran, dried beans and peas, fruits and psyllium fiber products are good sources of soluble fiber.

Starch: A type of complex carbohydrate found in foods like bread, pasta, rice, cereals, and starchy vegetables.

Stroke: Death of or damage to part of the brain caused by inadequate blood supply to the brain.

Systolic blood pressure: The higher number of a blood pressure reading, representing the force of blood against blood vessel walls as the heart beats.

Transient Ischemic Attacks: Temporary dizziness or loss of speech, vision or other body functions caused by inadequate or temporarily-blocked blood supply to part of the brain. Transient ischemic attacks often signal an impending stroke.

Triglycerides: The chemical storage form of fat in the body.

Vein: A blood vessel that carries blood from body tissues back to the heart

Very-low-density lipoprotein (VLDL): A type of lipoprotein that contains high levels of triglyceride and may also promote heart disease.

Whole-grain: A term referring to foods that are made from the entire grain kernel, including the high-fiber bran coating. Whole-grain foods include brown rice, oatmeal, pumpernickel or 100 percent whole wheat bread, and whole-grain cereals.

CHOLESTEROL IN FOODS

CHEESES

Blue cheese .... 1 oz. .... 21 mg.
Brie cheese .... 1 oz. .... 28 mg.
Cheddar cheese .... 1 oz. .... 30 mg.
Cream cheese .... 1 oz. .... 31 mg.
Cottage cheese, creamed .... 1/2 cup .... 17 mg.
Cottage cheese, dry curd .... 1/2 cup .... 5 mg.
Mozzarella cheese, (from whole milk) ...... 1 oz. .... 22 mg.
Mozzarella cheese, (from skim milk) .... 1 oz. .... 15 mg.
Swiss cheese .... 1 oz. .... 26 mg.

PROTEINS

Beef (3-1/2 ounces, cooked)

Corned, canned .... 85 mg.
Ground, regular .... 88 mg.
Liver, fried .... 478 mg.
Rib-eye, lean .... 75 mg.
Roast, rib .... 79 mg.
Roast, round .... 81 mg.

Eggs

Egg yolk .... 1 .... 274 mg.
Egg white .... 1 .... 0 mg.

Fish and Shellfish (3-1/2 ounces, cooked)

Clams .... 60 mg.
Cod .... 47 mg.
Crab .... 88 mg.
Flounder .... 68 mg.
Haddock .... 74 mg.
Halibut .... 58 mg.
Oysters .... 109 mg.
Shrimp .... 195 mg.
Trout, Rainbow .... 73 mg.
Tuna, canned .... 18 mg.

Pork (3-1/2 ounces, cooked)

Ham lunchmeat, extra lean .... 47 mg.
Ham steak, lean .... 54 mg.
Pork chops, lean .... 99 mg.
Ribroast, lean .... 78 mg.
Smoked link sausage .... 68 mg.
Bratwurst .... 60 mg.
Bacon.................................... 3 slices............... 16 mg.

Poultry (3-1/2 ounces, cooked)

Chicken, light meat, no skin .... 83 mg.
Chicken, dark meat, no skin .... 91 mg.
Duck, flesh only.. 87 mg.
Turkey, light meat, no skin.............................. 69 mg.
Turkey, dark meat, no skin .... 84 mg.

DESSERTS

Chocolate cake with frosting .... 1/16 cake .... 37 mg.
Cheesecake .... 1/12 cake .... 170 mg.
Danish pastry .... 1 .... 49 mg.
Caramels .... 1 oz. .... 1 mg.
Sherbet, orange .... 1/2 cup.................. 7 mg.

DAIRY PRODUCTS

Butter .... 1 tbsp. .... 31 mg.
Buttermilk .... 1 cup .... 9 mg.
Cream, half and half .... 1 tbsp. .... 6 mg.
Custard, baked .... 1 cup .... 278 mg.
Egg nog .... 1 cup .... 149 mg.
Ice cream, vanilla .... 1/2 cup .... 44 mg.
Ice milk, vanilla .... 1/2 cup .... 9 mg.
Milk, skim .... 1 cup .... 4 mg.
Milk, whole .... 1 cup .... 33 mg.
Milk, 1% fat .... 1 cup .... 10 mg.
Milk, 2% fat .... 1 cup .... 18 mg.
Pudding, vanilla .... 1/2 cup............... 15 mg.
Sour cream .... 1 tbsp. .... 6 mg.
Yogurt bar, plain .... 1 .... 5 mg.
Yogurt, low fat .... 1 cup.................... 4 mg.

SAUCES/SEASONINGS/DRESSINGS

Catsup .... 1 tbsp. .... 0 mg.
Cheese sauce .... 1/4 cup .... 13 mg.
Corn oil .... 1 tbsp. .... 0 mg.
French dressing .... 1 tbsp. .... 0 mg.
Hollandaise sauce .... 1/4 cup .... 13 mg.
Lard .... 1 tbsp. .... 12 mg.
Margarine .... 1 tbsp. .... 0 mg.
Mayonnaise .... 1 tbsp. .... 8 mg.
Salad dressing .... 1 tbsp. .... 4 mg.
Tartar sauce .... 1 tbsp. .... 4 mg.
Thousand Island dressing .... 1 tbsp. .... 4 mg.

BAKED GOODS

Bagel .... 1 .... 0 mg
Blueberry muffin .... 1 .... 32 mg.
Corn chips .... 1 oz. .... 0 mg.
Croissant .... 1 .... 13 mg.
Doughnut .... 1 .... 20 mg.
English muffin .... 1 .... 0 mg.
Pretzels .... 10 .... 0 mg.
Waffle .... 1 .... 81 mg.

FAST FOODS

ARBY'S

Roast Beef Sandwich.. 39 mg.
Jamocha shake .... 35 mg.

BURGER KING

Whopper.. 90 mg.
Whaler .... 77 mg.

DAIRY QUEEN

Cone, regular size... 15 mg.
Shake, regular size.. 50 mg.

HARDEE'S

Hamburger .... 20 mg.
Hot Ham and Cheese .... 68 mg.

JACK IN THE BOX

Taco Salad... 91 mg.
Supreme Crescent .... 178 mg.

TACO BELL

Burito Supreme .... 35 mg.
Taco Salad... 85 mg.

WENDY'S

Chili.. 30 mg.
Hamburger, single... 65 mg.

FAT CONTENT OF HIGH PROTEIN FOODS

FOOD	LOW FAT	MEDIUM FAT	HIGH FAT
Beef	Round (eye,top), sirloin, flank, chipped beef	Ground, roast (rib, chuck, rump), steak (cubed, Porterhouse, T-bone), meatloaf	Ribs, corned beef, prime rib
Pork	Fresh ham, tenderloin, Canadian bacon	Chops, loin, Boston butt, roast, cutlets	Spareribs, ground pork, sausage, bacon, country style ribs
Poultry	Chicken, turkey, Cornish hen		Fried chicken, poultry skin
Fish	Crab, clams, lobster, scallops, shrimp, oysters, sardines, smoked herring, water-packed tuna	Oil-packed tuna	Fried fish, fish sticks
Cheese	Cottage cheese	Diet cheeses, skim or part-skim milk cheeses, Ricotta, and Mozzarella	American, Blue, Brick, Brie, Cheddar, Cream, Edam, Feta, Gouda, Muenster, Parmesan, Provolone, Swiss
Other	95% fat free luncheon meat, egg whites, egg substitutes, dried beans and peas		Bologna, salami, pimento loaf, Knockwurst, Bratwurst, peanut butter, frankfurters, cashews, Macadamia nuts, peanuts, mixed nuts, pumpkin seeds, sesame seeds, sunflower seeds.

SMOKING CESSATION PROGRAMS

American Lung Association

Freedom from Smoking in 20 Days

A self-help manual offering step-by-step guidelines to help kick the smoking habit using behavior modification techniques.

A Lifetime of Freedom from Smoking

A maintenance manual for ex-smokers to help prevent backsliding.

Freedom from Smoking

A seven-week series of group sessions to help you quit smoking by examining why a person wants to quit and developing strategies.

In Control, A Video Freedom from Smoking Program

A thirteen segment series for individuals or groups to provide daily encouragement and motivation.

American Cancer Society

Seven-Day Plan to Help You Stop Smoking

A booklet that gives guidelines on quitting in a short time and tips to help along the way.

Freshstart

This program consists of four one-hour sessions to be viewed over two weeks and designed to give groups guidelines and support mechanisms to quit smoking.

National Cancer Institute

Staffs a toll-free number to provide information on smoking cessation programs nation-wide. CAll 1-800-4-CANCER.

Commercial

Smokenders

This is a six week behavior modification program stressing weight control, group support and motivational techniques. It is set up as a group program. For more information write to Smokenders, 50 Washington Street, Norwalk, CT 06854 or call 1-800-323-1126.

SAMPLE REGULAR HCF MEAL PLANS

1200 CALORIE MEAL PLAN

Breakfast

1	cup	cereal, Cheerios
3/4	cup	blueberries
1	cup	milk, skim
1/2		English muffin, whole grain
1	T.	margarine, light

Dinner

3	oz.	turkey breast, baked
1/2	cup	lima beans
1/2	cup	broccoli, chopped
1	small	roll, wheat
1	T.	margarine, light

Lunch

1	cup	lettuce, shredded
1/2	cup	carrots, diced
1/2	cup	zucchini, raw
1/2	med.	tomato, diced
2	T.	Italian dressing
4	slices	Melba Toast
1	cup	milk, skim

Snack

3	cups	popcorn, air-popped

1500 CALORIE MEAL PLAN

Breakfast

2		muffins, pineappple oat bran
2	T.	margarine, light
1	cup	vegetable juice

Dinner

4	oz.	pork chop, lean
1/2	cup	black-eyed peas
1	8" ear	corn
1	small	roll, rye
1	T.	margarine, light

Lunch

1		Peanut butter sandwich containing:
2	T.	peanut butter on
2	slices	bread, whole grain
1/2	med.	banana
1	cup	milk, skim

Snacks

15		grapes
1	cup	milk, skim

1800 CALORIE MEAL PLAN

Breakfast

2/3	cup	cereal, Common Sense
1	cup	milk, skim
1/2		bagel, toasted
1	T.	margarine, light
1/2	cup	apple juice

Lunch

1		Chicken sandwich with:
3	oz.	chicken, sliced
2	slices	bread, whole grain
1	leaf	lettuce
1/4		tomato, sliced
2	T.	margarine, light
1	small	apple
1	cup	milk, skim

Dinner

6	oz.	flounder, baked
1/2	cup	pinto beans
1	cup	Broccoli, Cauliflower and Mushroom Medley *
2/3	cup	rice
1		roll, rye
1	T.	margarine, light
3/4	cup	orange sections

Snacks

1/2		Pita Pocket with:
3/4	cup	Vegetarian sandwich filling *
1	med.	peach

2000 CALORIE MEAL PLAN

Breakfast

1	cup	cereal, Wheaties
1	cup	milk, skim
1		muffin, oat bran
1	T.	margarine, light
1	cup	juice, grapefruit

Lunch

1		Ham and Cheese sandwich with:
2	oz.	ham, lean
1	oz.	cheese, low-calorie
2	slices	bread, whole grain
2	T.	salad dressing, low-calorie
1/2	cup	carrot sticks
1/4	med.	avocado
1	med.	pear

Dinner

4	ounce	beef, flank steak
1/2	cup	Seasoned Beans *
1	small	potato, baked
3	t.	margarine, light
1/2	cup	peas, green
1/2	cup	carrots
1/2	cup	applesauce, unsweetened

Snacks

1/2	cup	cereal, Raisin Squares
1	cup	milk, skim
2	squares	graham cracker
1		orange

*   These recipes are found in **THE HCF GUIDE BOOK**.

SAMPLE AGGRESSIVE HCF MEAL PLANS

1200 CALORIE AGGRESSIVE HCF MEAL PLAN

Breakfast

5	oz.	Fruited Yogurt *
1		muffin, oat bran
1	T.	margarine, light

Lunch

1/4	cup	tuna, water-pack
4	slices	toast, melba
2	T.	salad dressing, low-calorie
8	small	olives, green
1/2	cup	celery sticks
1		nectarine

Dinner

1/2	cup	lima beans
1	small	potato, baked
1/2	cup	carrots
1	cup	Tossed Salad *
2	T.	French dressing, low-calorie
1		apple

Snack

2/3	cup	Oat Flakes
1	cup	milk, skim
2	T.	raisins

1500 CALORIE AGGRESSIVE HCF MEAL PLAN

Breakfast

3/4	cup	oatmeal
2	T.	raisins
1/2	cup	milk, skim

Lunch

1		Stuffed Green Pepper *
1/2	cup	cabbage
1		muffin, oat bran
2	T.	margarine, light
1		nectarine
1/2	cup	milk, skim

Dinner

3	oz.	swordfish
1/2	cup	spinach
1/2	small	sweet potato
3	T.	margarine, light
1	cup	fruit salad

Snacks

12		cherries
1	cup	milk, skim
4		graham crackers
1-1/2	t.	peanut butter

*   These recipes are found in the **HCF GUIDE BOOK**.

1800 CALORIE AGGRESSIVE HCF MEAL PLAN

Breakfast

2		Oatmeal Pancakes *
2	T.	margarine, light
3/4	cup	blueberries
3/4	cup	oat bran
1	cup	milk, skim

Lunch

1	cup	Navy bean soup
1		muffin, oat bran
1	T.	margarine, light
1		apple

Dinner

4	oz.	Flounder Fillet *
2/3	cup	rice, brown
1	cup	beans, green
1	med.	tomato, sliced
3/4	cup	pineapple
1		muffin, oat bran
2	T.	margarine, light

Snacks

1	med.	banana
2/3	cup	cereal, Common Sense
1	cup	milk, skim

2000 CALORIE AGGRESSIVE HCF MEAL PLAN

Breakfast

2/3	cup	Granola Cereal **
1	cup	milk, skim
1		muffin, oat bran
15		grapes
1	cup	grapefruit juice

Lunch

1/2	cup	cottage cheese, dry curd
1	med.	tomato, sliced
2	T.	salad dressing, low-calorie
1		muffin, oat bran
1	T.	margarine, light
2	med.	plums

Dinner

1-1/2	cup	Chili *
1/4	cup	onion, chopped
1/2	cup	green peppers, chopped
6	squares	crackers, rye
1		pear
1	cup	milk, skim

Snacks

1/4	cup	Party Shrimp Spread *
1/2	cup	cauliflower, raw
4		toast points, whole grain
15		pistachios
1	cup	raspberries
3/4	cup	blueberries

---

*   These recipes are found in the **HCF GUIDE BOOK.**
** These recipes are found in **DR. ANDERSON'S LIFE-SAVING DIET.**

METROPOLITAN WEIGHT TABLES

DESIRABLE WEIGHTS FOR MEN AND WOMEN, AGES 25 AND OVER, ACCORDING TO HEIGHT AND FRAME*

Men: Weight in Pounds (indoor clothing)

Height (in shoes)**	Small Frame	Medium Frame	Large Frame
5'2"	112 - 120	118 - 129	126 - 141
5'3"	115 - 123	121 - 133	129 - 144
5'4"	118 - 126	124 - 136	132 - 148
5'5"	121 - 129	127 - 139	135 - 152
5'6"	124 - 133	130 - 143	138 - 156
5'7"	128 - 137	134 - 147	142 - 161
5'8"	132 - 141	138 - 152	147 - 166
5'9"	136 - 145	142 - 156	151 - 170
5'10"	140 - 150	146 - 160	155 - 174
5'11"	144 - 154	150 - 165	159 - 179
6'0"	148 - 158	154 - 170	164 - 184
6'1"	152 - 162	158 - 175	168 - 189
6'2"	156 - 167	162 - 180	173 - 194
6'3"	160 - 171	167 - 185	178 - 199
6'4"	164 - 175	172 - 190	182 - 204

Women: Weight in Pounds (indoor clothing)

Height (in shoes)	Small Frame	Medium Frame	Large Frame
4'10"	92 - 98	96 - 107	104 - 119
4'11"	94 - 101	98 - 110	106 - 122
5'0"	96 - 104	101 - 113	109 - 125
5'1"	99 - 107	104 - 116	112 - 128
5'2"	102 - 110	107 - 119	115 - 131
5'3"	105 - 113	110 - 122	118 - 134
5'4"	108 - 116	113 - 126	121 - 138
5'5"	111 - 119	116 - 130	125 - 142
5'6"	114 - 123	120 - 135	129 - 146
5'7"	118 - 127	124 - 139	133 - 150
5'8"	122 - 131	128 - 143	137 - 154
5'9"	126 - 135	132 - 147	141 - 158
5'10"	130 - 140	136 - 151	145 - 163
5'11"	134 - 144	140 - 155	149 - 168
6'0"	138 - 148	144 - 159	153 - 173

* *Prepared by the Metropolitan Life Insurance Company. Derived primarily from data of the Build and Blood Pressure Study, 1959, Society of Actuaries.*

** *Allow 1" heels for men's shoes and 2" heels for women's shoes.*

COOKBOOKS

American Heart Association Cookbook. 4th edition, edited by Ruth Eshleman, Ed.D. and Mary Winston, R.D. David McKay Co., Inc., New York, 1984.

Diet for a Small Planet. Frances Moore Lappe. Ballantine Books. New York, 1982.

New York Times New Natural Foods Cookbook. New York Times Book Co., New York, 1982.

The New American Diet. Sonja L. Connor, M.S., R.D. and William E. Connor, M.D. Simon and Schuster, New York, 1986.

Vegetarian. Nava Atlas. Dial Press. Doubleday and Co., Garden City, New York, 1984.

Recipes for a Small Planet. Ellen Buchman Ewald. Ballantine Books, New York, 1973.

American Wholefoods Cuisine. Nikki and David Goldberg. New American Library, New York, 1983.

The Los Angeles Times Natural Foods Cookbook. Jeanne Voltz, Signet Book, 1975.

Family Cookbooks, Vols. I, II, and III. American Diabetes Association/American Dietetic Association, Prentice-Hall, Englewood Cliffs, N.J.

Don't Eat Your Heart Out Cookbook. Joseph C. Piscatela, Workman Publishing Co., New York, 1987.

Dr. Anderson's Life-Saving Diet. James W. Anderson, M.D., The Body Press, 1986. Distributed by The HCF Nutrition Research Foundation Inc., P.O. Box 22124, Lexington, KY. 40522, (606) 276-3119.

READING MATERIALS

SMOKING CESSATION

No More Butts. A Psychologist's Approach to Quitting Cigarettes. Richard W. Olshavsky. Indiana University Press, Bloomington, IN 1977.

Quit Smoking. Curtis Casewit. Para Research, Inc., Rockport, MA 1983.

Switch Down and Quit. Dolly D. Gahagan. Ten Speed Press, 1987.

EXERCISE

Surviving Exercise. Judy Alter. Houghton Mifflin, Co., Inc. Boston, 1983.

The Aerobics Way. Kenneth H. Cooper, M.D. M. Evans and Company, Inc., New York, 1977.

Aerobic Dancing. Jackie Sorensen. Rawson, Wade Publishers, Inc., New York, 1979.

The Athlete's Kitchen. Nancy Clark. New England Sports Publications, P.O. Box 252 Boston, Ma. 02113, 1981

HYPERTENSION

Managing Hypertension. James W. Warren, and Genell J. Subak-Sharpe. Doubleday and Company, Inc.. Garden City, New York, 1986.

Understanding Hypertension. Timothy N. Caris. Warner Books, New York, 1985.

Coping With High Blood Pressure. Sandy Sorrention and Carl Hausman Red Dembner Enterprises Co., New York, 1986.

Control Your High Blood Pressure Without Drugs. Cleaves M. Bennet, M.D. Doubleday and Co., Inc. Garden City, New York, 1984.

Salt-Free Cookbook. Ruth Baum and Hilary Baum. Putnam Publishing Group, New York, 1985.

STRESS

Stress, Diet and Your Heart. Dean Ornish. Holt, Rinehart and Winston. New York, 1982.

Type A Behavior and Your Heart. Meyer Friedman and Ray Rosenman. Knopf. New York, 1974.

Birkam's Beginning Yoga Class. Birkam Choudhury. J.P Tarcher, Inc. Los Angeles, 1978.

Is It Worth Dying For? Robert S. Eliot, M.D. and Dennis L. Breo. Bantam Books, New York, 1984.

Stress and the Art of Biofeedback. Barbara A. Brown. Harper and Row. New York, 1977.

NUTRITION

The HCF Guide Book. James W. Anderson, M.D., HCF Nutrition Research Foundation, P.O. Box 22124, Lexington, KY 40522, 1987.

Cooking A'La Heart. Mankato Heart Health Program. Mankato Heart Health Program Foundation, Inc., 101 North Second Street, Suite 202, Mankato, MN 56001,1988.

Adding Fiber to Your Diet. Park Nicollet Medical Foundation. DCI Publishing Diabetes Center, Inc., Post Office # 739. Wayzata, MN 55391.

Dr. Anderson's Life-Saving Diet. James W. Anderson, M.D. The Body Press, Tucson, AZ, 1984.

The Living Heart Diet. Michael DeBakey, M.D. Simon and Schuster, New York, 1984.

Heart Health

Recovering from the Heart Attack Experience. Elizabeth Weiss. Macmillan Publishing Co., Inc. New York, 1980.

The Pritikin Program for Diet and Exercise. Nathan Pritikin. Grosset and Dunlap. New York, 1979.

Heart Talk, Preventing and Coping with Silent and Painful Heart Disease Peter F. Cohn, M.D. and Joan K. Cohn, M.D. Harcourt, Brace, Jovanovich, New York, 1987.

The American Medical Association Book of Heart Care. American Medical Association. Random House, New York, 1982.

RECIPES

BEAN SPREAD

16	oz.	pinto beans
10	oz.	whole tomatoes and green chilies
1/8	t.	pepper
1	dash	tabasco sauce

Rinse and drain beans; mash well. Add all the tomatoes and 1/2 of the juice from the whole tomatoes and green chilies. Add pepper and tabasco sauce and stir. Bake in 350 degree oven for 20 minutes. Serve with low fat crackers or use as a filling in bean burritos.

Yield: 1 cup (1/4 cup per serving)
Exchanges Per Serving: 1 Bean
Kcal 112, CHO 20 g., PRO 8 g., FAT 0 , FIBER 5 g.

9 BEAN SOUP

9	cup	beans, different varieties (use different colors to add variety)
4	oz.	ham
1	large	onion, chopped
1	clove	garlic, minced
		seasonings to taste
1	can (28 oz.)	whole tomatoes, chopped
1	can (16 oz.)	tomatoes and green chilies, chopped.

Cover beans with water and soak overnight. Drain and rinse beans and put in a large pot with hms. Add the onion, garlic and seasonings to tast Cook 3-4 hours or in a crock pot all day. Add the tomatoes and green chilies and cook 30-40 minutes longer.

Yield: 9 servings. (2 cups per serving)
Exchanges Per Serving: 2 Beans, 1 Garden Vegetable
Kcal 240, CHO 40 g., PRO 19 g., FAT 1 g., FIBER 12 g.

SEAFOOD PASTA SALAD

12	oz.	rainbow twirls, cooked and drained
1		bell pepper, chopped
1	small	onion, chopped
10	oz.	mushrooms, sliced
2		tomatoes, chopped
1-1/2	oz.	black olives, pitted and sliced
1/4	cup	Parmesan cheese
1	cup	celery, chopped
1	bottle (8 oz.)	No-Oil Italian dressing
1	lb.	imitation crab meat flakes

Combine all ingredients, mix well with dressing. Refrigerate until ready to serve.

Yield: 6 servings (2 cups per serving)
Exchanges Per Serving: 3 Starch, 1-1/2 Protein, 1 Garden Vegetable
Kcal 310, CHO 50 g., PRO 19 g., FAT 3 g., FIBER 8 g.

STEAMED RED SNAPPER WITH WINE & LEMON

1	lb.	red snapper fillets
4	slices	lemon
3/4	cup	onion, chopped
1/4	cup	wine, dry white
1	t.	lemon rind, grated
1/4	t.	pepper
2	T.	fresh parsley, chopped

In a 12" x 8" baking dish arrange fillets in a single layer. Top evenly with remaining ingredients. Cover loosely with wax paper; microwave on HIGH 4-7 minutes or until fish flakes easily when tested with a fork.

Yield: 4 servings (4 oz. per serving)
Exchanges Per Serving: 2 Protein
Kcal 135, CHO 2 g., PRO 16 g., FAT 3 g., FIBER .6 g.

FISH SEASONINGS

2	T.	dehydrated onion, minced
8	t.	dill weed
4	t.	garlic powder
4	t.	parsley flakes
2	t.	thyme
1	t.	paprika
1	t.	bay leaf powder
1/2	t.	tarragon
1/2	t.	dill seed
1/2	t.	savory

In a blender, blend dehydrated onion into fine pieces. Add remaining herbs. Blend to mix well but do not make into a powder. To keep herbs fresh, store in shaker top bottle with tight fitting lid.

Yield: 1-1/2 oz.

TOFU SPAGHETTI

1	pkg. (14 oz.)	Tofu, cubed
2	T.	olive oil
1/2	lbs.	mushrooms, sliced
1		green pepper, sliced
1	large	onion, sliced
1	jar (1 lb., 15-3/4 oz.)	Prego sauce, plain
1	can (2-1/4 oz.)	ripe olives, sliced
1	lb.	spaghetti, cooked

Chop tofu into small squares. Heat oil in skillet. Saute tofu and remove from pan. Saute sliced mushrooms, green pepper and onion. Add tofu, olives and Prego sauce and heat until warm. Pour over cooked spaghetti.

Yield: 6 servings
Exchanges Per Serving: 1 Starch, 1/2 Protein, 2 Garden Vegetables, 1 Fat
Kcal 226, CHO 38 g., PRO 10 g., FAT 9 g., FIBER 7 g.

OAT BREAD

1/3	cup	oats, dry
2	T.	margarine
2	T.	honey
1	t.	salt (optional)
3/4	cup	boiling water
1	T.	active dry yeast
1/2	t.	sugar
1/2	cup	hot water
2	cups	whole wheat flour, sifted
1	cup	oat bran, dry
2		egg whites

Preheat oven to 375°. Put oats, margarine, honey, salt and boiling water in large bowl. Stir to mix well. Set aside and allow to cool. Sprinkle yeast and 1/2 teaspoon sugar over hot water. Stir to dissolve yeast. Let stand until mixture bubbles, 5-10 minutes. Sift whole wheat flour and remeasure. Place oat bran in blender and blend a few minutes. Mix flour and oat bran together. Set aside.

Stir cooled oat bran mixture, dissolved yeast mixture and egg whites together. Using an electric mixer, preferably a large mixer as opposed to a hand held, gradually add flour and oat bran mixture. Mix about two minutes. Spoon mixture, which will be very stiff, into a prepared 9"x5"x3" loaf pan. Prepare pan by using a vegetable spray or lightly oiling. Loosely cover baking pan with wax paper and a towel. Place in a warm spot, away from drafts and allow to rise for approximately 75 minutes. Bake in pre-heated oven for 50-60 minutes or until bread is done. Loaf should sound hollow when thumped or knife should come out clean. Allow to cool a few minutes. Cut out of pan gently.

Yield: 1 loaf, approximately 20 slices. Serving = 1 slice.

Exchanges Per Serving: 1 Starch

Kcal 80, CHO 15 g., PRO 2 g., FAT 1 g., FIBER 2 g.

ARTICHOKE PARMESAN DIP

1	can (14 oz.)	artichoke hearts
1/4	cup	salad dressing, light
1	cup	parmesan cheese
1/3	cup	oat bran, dry

Preheat oven to 350°. Drain artichoke hearts. Save the liquid. Chop into small pieces. Mix all ingredients together. Add enough artichoke liquid to moisten mixture. Bake in 350° oven for 15-20 minutes or until mixture bubbles. Serve hot or cold with whole wheat crackers.

Yield: 2 cups (2 tablespoons per serving)

Exchanges per serving: ½ Vegetable, ½ Protein

Kcal 45, CHO 2 g., PRO 4 g., FAT 2 g., FIBER .5 g.

PINEAPPLE MUFFINS

2	cup	oat bran, dry
1/2	cup	flour, white all-purpose
1/4	cup	brown sugar
1	T.	baking powder
1/2	cup	milk, skim
1	can	pineapple, crushed in juice (unsweetened)
2		egg substitute
2	T.	vegetable oil

Preheat oven to 425 degrees. Mix the oat bran, flour, brown sugar and baking powder in a bowl. Mix the milk, pineapple with juice, egg substitute and oil in a large bowl. Add the dry ingredients and mix just until moistened. Spray muffin pans with pan coating. Fill muffin cups 2/3 full with batter and bake for 17 minutes.

Yield: 12 muffins. (1 muffin per serving)
Exchanges Per Serving: 1/2 Fat, 1/2 Cereal
Kcal 118, CHO 21 g., PRO 3 g., FAT 3 g., FIBER 3 g.

APPLE CINNAMON MUFFINS

2	cups	oat bran, dry
1/2	cup	flour, white all-purpose
1/4	cup	brown sugar or honey
1	T.	baking powder
1-1/4	t.	cinnamon
3/4	cup	apple juice
1/2	cup	milk, skim
2		egg substitute
2	T.	vegetable oil
1	medium	apple, chopped

Optional (add calories and exchanges)

1/4	cup	chopped nuts (2 Fats)
1/4	cup	raisins (2 Fruit)

Preheat oven to 425 degrees. Mix the oat bran, flour, brown sugar, baking powder and cinnamon in a small bowl. Mix the apple juice, milk, egg substitute and vegetable oil in a large bowl. Stir in the dry ingredients and apple, mixing until just moistened. Spray the muffin tins with pan coating. Fill muffin cups 2/3 full with batter and bake for 17 minutes.

Yield: 12 muffins. (1 muffin per serving)
Exchanges Per Serving: 1/2 Fat, 1/2 Cereal
Kcal 129, CHO 22 g., PRO 4 g., FAT 3 g., FIBER 3 g.

ORANGE FISH FILLETS

1	lb.	orange roughy
2	T.	orange juice concentrate
1	T.	lemon juice
1/2	t.	dill weed, dried
1/2	t.	fish seasonings
1	T.	parsley, finely chopped
1/4	cup	water
2	T.	sesame seeds, toasted

Place fish in a glass casserole. Combine orange juice concentrate, lemon juice, dill weed, fish seasonings, parsley and water, pouring these over the fish. Cover and marinate in refrigerator 45 minutes, turning once. Preheat the broiler. Place marinated fish on a broiler pan sprayed with pan coating. Broil four inches from the heat until fish flakes, about 10-15 minutes. Baste often with marinade. Serve with heated marinade and toasted sesame seeds.

Yield: 4 servings (4 oz. per serving)
Exchanges Per Serving: 2 Protein, 1 Fat
Kcal 141, CHO 2 g., PRO 16 g., FAT 8 g., FIBER 0

TOMATO FLOUNDER

2	small	onions, sliced
2	T.	margarine
1	clove	garlic, finely chopped
1	can (16 oz)	stewed tomatoes, chopped
1	cup	mushrooms, sliced
1/4	cup	white wine
1/8	t.	basil
		salt
6	1/4 lb. fillets	flounder

Microwave Directions

In oblong baking dish, combine onion, margarine and garlic; heat, covered, 3 to 3 1/2 minutes on HIGH. Stir in tomatoes, mushrooms, wine and basil. Heat, covered 3 minutes on HIGH. Continue cooking on MEDIUM HIGH an additional 3 to 4 minutes. Arrange fish seam-side down in sauce; spoon sauce over the fish. Heat, covered, 5 to 6 minutes on HIGH until fish is done. Let stand, covered, 5 minutes before serving.

Yield: 6 servings (4 oz.)
Exchanges Per Serving: 2 Protein, 1 Garden Vegetable, 1 Fat
Kcal 177, CHO 4 g., PRO 17 g., FAT 9 g., FIBER 2 g.

PUBLICATIONS OF THE HCF NUTRITION RESEARCH FOUNDATION, INC.

DIABETES AND NUTRITION NEWS. Quarterly newsletter from Dr. Anderson and his team concerning pertinent facts for living healthy lives, the latest in research, and new publications. (*Available in U.S. only*).

THE HCF GUIDE BOOK (1987). "How to" for HCF Plan. This user's guide to the HCF diet lists specifics and practical suggestions for today's pace and lifestyle.

HCF EXCHANGES: A SENSIBLE PLAN FOR HEALTHY EATING (1987). Companion to Guide Book - Listing of the HCF exchange groups and daily meal plan for health professionals to prescribe a specific calorie level.

NUTRITION MANAGEMENT OF METABOLIC CONDITIONS (1988). Updated comprehensive professional manual on rationale and specifics for using high fiber diets for diabetes, obesity, hypoglycemia and hyperlipidemia.
Update only (1988) Revised appendix to update your professional guide.

PLANT FIBER IN FOODS (1986). A fiber reference manual. Total fiber as well as soluble fiber content of 300+ foods. Values listed in grams and portion sizes.

DIABETES: A PRACTICAL GUIDE TO HEALTHY LIVING (1983). An excellent guide for general diabetes management written by Dr. Anderson, with a special section on the HCF diet plan.

DR. ANDERSON'S LIFE-SAVING DIET (1986). Meal plans, recipes and tips for eating the high fiber, high carbohydrate, low fat way to keep slim and healthy.

HCF LIFESTYLE RECORD BOOK (1988). A daily intake record book for 30 days that explains the HCF Way to better health. It can be used in the treatment of diabetes, heart disease, weight reduction, etc.

HCF FIBER FACTS (1988). A pocket sized booklet summarizing the facts on fiber and listing high fiber sources by exchanges.

For more information and current pricing contact

HCF Nutrition Research Foundation, Inc.
P. O. Box 22124
Lexington, KY 40522
(606) 276-3119